THE HABITAT AFFECT

Anna Cherry

THE HABITAT AFFECT – 2nd EDITION

Copyright © 2017 Anna Cherry

All rights reserved. No part of this publication may be reproduced, stored in a retrieval system, or transmitted in any form or by any means, electronic, mechanical, photocopying, recording or otherwise, without the prior consent of the copyright owner.

DISCLAIMER: The content of The Habitat Affect is for general information only and is not intended to be a substitute for professional advice or treatment. No warranties, guarantees, promises or representations, express or implied, concerning the content accuracy, completeness, timeliness or usefulness of any opinions, advice or other information contained or referenced in this book, are made. In consideration of your use and access to this book, you agree that in no event will any party involved in creating, producing or delivering The Habitat Affect book, or any website or social media platform linked to this publication, be liable to you in any manner whatsoever for any decision made or action or non-action taken by you in reliance upon the information provided herein. Please note that by reading this book, you agree to be bound by these terms and conditions. If you do not wish to be so bound, you should not engage with The Habitat Affect nor use the 9 Enrichments Experience self-development system.

habitataffect.com

facebook.com/AnnaCosmicCherry

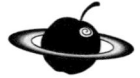

PUBLISHED by Cosmic Cherry

COVER DESIGN by Sally Hughes

ISBN: 978-1-9998497-0-2

THE HABITAT AFFECT

How to use your home surroundings and your mental-emotional experiences to enrich your life and the lives of all those with whom you connect.

Create your individual Habitat Affect by engaging with the 9 Enrichments Experience which draws on the insights of psychology, bioscience, buddhist philosophy, mindfulness, fitness and health. Introducing Focus Features: highly-personal physical cues around your home to motivate and inspire you.

Join us for a life-changing journey around your physical, mental and emotional environments. There are no rigid rules, simply suggestions and fresh ideas to help guide your individual choices-for-change and new experiences.

When we choose differently – we create differently.

Author's note: the noun 'affect' is used in psychology to describe a factor influencing behaviour. Herein it refers to the psychological influences of the stimuli in our surroundings – our 'habitat' – on our senses and thinking, from which flow our behaviour and everyday experiences.

CONTENTS

Prologue

Part 1: Overture to your renewal 1

1. Setting the scene 2
2. Scope of the 9 Enrichments 9
3. Sensual clutter-free settings 18
4. The power of colour and plants 26
5. Your life in the round 31
6. Understanding your choices. 39
7. Health and your body 49
8. Mind matters – luck – 100% now 57
9. Actions speak louder than words 66

Part 2: Experiencing the habitat affect 71

1st Enrichment Experience 72
2nd Enrichment Experience. 85
3rd Enrichment Experience 99
4th Enrichment Experience 108
5th Enrichment Experience 118
6th Enrichment Experience 151
7th Enrichment Experience 165
8th Enrichment Experience 176
9th Enrichment Experience 192

Sustaining an enriched way of life 207

CONTENTS cont.

Appendix 219

A: Colour attributes 220

B: Dealing with fears, doubts and worry 226

C: Inside the elements 235

D: Mindfulness practice – an overview 237

E: Ready to receive 240

F: Keeping love alive 242

G: Appreciating the miracle of me 245

H: Foods that affect your vitality 248

I: Developing your listening skills 250

J: From flour to flourishing 253

K: Reality and your choices 255

L: Compass and element chart 256

M: The 5 elements 257

About the Author

DEDICATION

This book is dedicated to my four amazing children – Georgia, Chloe, Jemma and Justin – who enrich my life enormously and are a constant source of delight.

Your home is a unique reflection of yourself – from the way you arrange it and the décor you choose, to the many items you place in it. With fresh insight, you can easily adjust your surroundings to support your life goals and enhance your well-being.

PROLOGUE

Have you ever asked yourself how the place where you live affects your life? How does your home, the type of building, the rooms, the open spaces, the stuff you hold onto, impact the quality of your experiences? Equally, how do the places you visit in your mind – your daily thoughts and feelings – influence the quality of your choices and decisions, and hence your enjoyment of life?

We are living through extraordinarily confusing times: fast-evolving technologies, climate change, international terrorism, financial uncertainty, body image fascination and obsessive celebrity culture. New technologies and modern conveniences are designed to make our lives easier, yet the reality is that many of us are actually feeling overwhelmed, busier, more anxious, restless, joyless and discontent. Even if you are reasonably happy and comfortable, perhaps you are reading this because you feel like something isn't quite right in your life. You may be questioning your core values and trying to decide what is really important to you, to those you love and to the planet.

The Habitat Affect is designed to lead you on a path of personal realisation and wise choices so that you can build an inspirational set of life practices for the benefit of all. To do this, we invite you to explore both your physical self and your mental-emotional mindscape in unison. Your home – whether it be a small apartment or a large house – represents the tangible foundation on which your everyday vitality is nurtured, and from which you go out to face the world. Inseparably, your mental environment – thoughts, attitudes and emotions, and the way you make decisions – impacts all your experiences.

In Part 1 we introduce you to the principles of the Habitat Affect as you embark on a journey of self-discovery and openness to change. We suggest you take a critical look at your current mental and physical environs and how they might affect you – from hindering clutter to calm order, from bad habits to vibrant well-being, from your doubts and worries to colour and sunlight. By being consciously aware of your power to choose helpful essentials for your life – on purpose – you can create the causes and conditions in which to learn and grow and manifest your dreams.

In Part 2 you create your own personal Habitat Affect through experiencing the 9 Enrichments which are drawn from a vast canon of psychology, bioscience, Buddhism, mindfulness, health, fitness and Feng Shui, and cover just about every area of your life. You will be motivated to take responsibility for making choices-for-change which can be honoured with physical Focus Features around your home. These evident features – design concepts, décor and placements, will act as daily reminders to direct your energy wherever it is needed – your career, your relationships, your body and health, your ability to overcome difficulties, to learn and to finish projects, your finances, your confidence, self-respect and sanctuary.

By making appropriate changes – radical or subtle – to your physical surroundings alongside addressing your stresses and delights, we strongly believe you will be better equipped to flourish in today's frenetic world and, by example, enrich the lives of all those with whom you connect.

Anna Cherry & Chloe Roberts © 2017

PART 1

OVERTURE TO YOUR RENEWAL

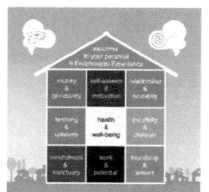

1. SETTING THE SCENE

"To find life's purpose we must go through the door of ourselves." In the spirit of this demanding quote from Krishnamurti, welcome to The Habitat Affect and the 9 Enrichments Experience. By interpreting the suggestions in this book to suit your personal circumstances you can create opportunities for life-changing experiences.

What is the Habitat Affect?

We use the term 'Affect' to refer to the psychological influence of the stimuli in our surroundings – our 'Habitat' – on our senses, our thinking and our emotional experiences from which flow our motivation and subsequent behaviour.

The 'Affect' we experience from our 'Habitat' can be high, neutral or low in its intensity to motivate us. Motivation is the impulsion to either do something or refrain from doing something – to take action or deliberate non-action. And, as we know only too well, motivation is a key driver in how we function and experience life.

As far as is humanly possible, if we strive to maintain 'balanced' self-control with regard to our attitudes and feelings, we can create an optimal state for motivating ourselves to live happy healthy lives. In this context, our motivation and behaviour, and hence our psychological well-being, is deeply influenced – affected – by our interactive relationship with the places we inhabit.

Naturally your well-being is dependent on more than just how you relate to your immediate habitat. It is, to a great extent, determined by your existing physical, mental and emotional makeup and attitudes – your genetic inherited characteristics and your learned knowledge, skills and behaviour.

Before considering specific things you can do to increase the supportive aspects of your habitat via the 9 Enrichments Experience [in Part 2], you are invited [later in Part 1] to review the context of your life in general – your individual circumstances and character, your attitudes, anxieties and aspirations – all of which make you 'the person you are today' – the person making the choices-for-change. Now a little more about the Habitat Affect itself.

'At home' with Environmental Psychology

The Habitat Affect has evolved from an area of Environmental Psychology specifically relating to your home and your workplace. Environmental Psychology is the study of the relationship between a given environment and the behaviour of its inhabitants; it focuses on the 'interplay' between people and their surroundings. In the context of the Habitat Affect, we are mainly concerned with the built environment – our human-made residences and their immediate surroundings.

Most of us identify with certain habitats in our lives, so it makes sense to see how they affect our behaviour. We can have an array of feelings, some subconscious, associated with significant places from our past or in our present. Feelings can range from total comfort to extreme discomfort, contentment with the familiar versus the excitement of the new. The influence of habitat can extend to our general attitude, the ability to generate ideas, the poignancy of memory, our personal values and preferences.

Is your environment really so important?

Yes – the psychological affect of your 'living conditions' is a key component of your well-being. Living in an environment that is aesthetically pleasing, comfortable and appropriately organised to suit your particular preferences is incredibly helpful. Living in an environment that is ugly, cluttered, uncomfortable and disorganised can be extremely hindering to your well-being. In this respect, you deserve to live and to work in places that are positively supportive.

In developed societies, we all live in buildings – our homes – whether it be a small flat or a large house. Picture yours for a moment in your mind's eye – how does it make you feel – does it make your heart sing? Some of us also spend a fair amount of time working in buildings. If that is you, picture yourself for a moment in your mind's eye in your workplace – how does it make you feel – does it make your heart sing?

Unhelpful environments

If you are still a little sceptical, just imagine the negative obstructions of living in a highly cluttered household. Worse still is the tension caused by noise pollution – living under a flight path, beside a main road or next to a railway; sharing a bed with a loud snorer; the sound of rowdy neighbours through partition walls; the deep beat of a rock concert. Whatever your personal experience, there is bound to be a noise or two that 'gets on your nerves'!

Other environmental factors which may have an adverse impact on mood include urban crowding, lack of access to natural daylight, garish colours, traffic pollution worries, unpleasant smells, damp and mould. On the other hand, a positively pleasing environment can be totally uplifting.

External environment – emotional environment

As well as our buildings, we are all surrounded by an external environment of some kind – not necessarily of our choosing but nonetheless the one within which we learn to cope and potentially hope to thrive. We can also take trips to visit other environments to enjoy things that we don't find at home – from the gym to extended periods away for holidays and sometimes for work projects.

Using the word 'environment' in its broadest sense, you can also think about your individual 'emotional environment', particularly as you learn more about the 9 Enrichments. For now, we hope you agree that you need a clear uncluttered mind to allow for wise elegant thoughts, emotional stability and the aptitude to turn good intentions into actions.

Creating environments that nurture your life force energy

In the Habitat Affect we are mindful of the eastern concept of Chi, Ki, or Qi, Prana in India – various words given to the vital life force energy. Chi is likened to an essential battery that makes the difference between your physical body being 'dead' or being 'alive'. Do a big stretch first thing in the morning and feel the energy coursing through your body.

Our life force energy is what distinguishes us, for example, from a stone, a plastic bag or a wind turbine – anything that appears to have no 'life force' energy. However, as physics has revealed, which we discuss later in this book, even the atoms of apparently 'lifeless' structures comprise perpetual energy in motion – everything interconnects and has the ability to influence us in subtle ways.

Therefore, our aim is always to live in harmony with our personal surroundings in order to nurture our life force energy and support its vital power to refresh mind and body.

Making the best of your living conditions

While there are generally constraints on where we live and the type of building we can afford, we can still make the best of what we have.

The primary decision about geographical location – where to live – is generally dictated by our circumstances, be it job prospects, financial considerations, relationship dynamics, parenting responsibilities, cultural influences, social norms and even wanderlust.

Likewise, the range of human dwellings is vast – from caves, mud huts and fortresses to tower blocks, luxury apartments, condominiums, country houses, beach dwellings, and everything in between.

Your personal type of residence is most likely dependent on your financial circumstances, your responsibility for housing other family members [children or an elderly parent], and your aesthetic tastes. Fortunately, whether your home is large or small, dark or light, enclosed or open, improvements can always be made.

Addressing your psychological influences

Whatever your type of home, the Habitat Affect is not just about moving a few objects around, painting the walls a different colour or shifting the furniture. To initiate powerful long-lasting results, we also ask you to visit your innermost thoughts regarding any areas of your life which you feel are currently unsatisfactory – where deep down you know there is room for change and improvement.

Once identified, these 'psychological areas' can be linked to 'physical areas' in your home to help you sustain wise choices in the future.

Intertwining the psychological and the physical

As part of the choices-for-change process, we invite you to participate in the 9 Enrichments Experience [Part 2]. This includes guidance on how to match your personal aspirations with specific rooms and spaces, providing a focus for whatever you wish to bring into being.

Within these recognised areas, you can clear the clutter, reorganise the space to suit your personal requirements, including colour aspects, and make physical placements which we call Focus Features to act as daily reminders of your intentions.

Whether Focus Features work by placebo effect or by other motivational means is open to question, but they do seem to provide fresh incentives and herald new opportunities.

Whatever the psychological mechanisms at work here, we maintain that by adapting certain aspects of your home to encourage your personal Habitat Affect, you will enjoy better 'living conditions' and enhance your life experiences.

An added benefit of using your surroundings to help sustain wise choices-for-change is that your renewed goodwill can issue a ripple effect with the potential to enrich the lives of those with whom you come into contact. Such benevolent communication with other people is the true source of your own happiness and a life well-lived.

Wise words

While you are re-discovering yourself and your environment, you might like to choose some supportive sayings and maxims that happen to resonate with you – they can have a potent influence on your thinking.

There is no shortage of wise words to inspire you – from your childhood, from books, from friends or via the internet

– enjoy discovering them and feeling their meaning for you personally. Maybe keep a 'sayings journal' or display them around your home and workplace as an aide memoire.

You will find a few of our favourite sayings scattered around this book. Here is one for openers attributed to Daniel Day-Lewis: *"I live in a landscape which, every single day of my life, is enriching."*

2. SCOPE OF THE 9 ENRICHMENTS

"I wanted to change the world. But I have found that the only thing one can be sure of changing is oneself." Aldous Huxley. In a sense, your home habitat is a reflection of the inner you. This 'inner you' is a wonderfully complex mix of your inherited nature, your upbringing, your adult experiences and the current circumstances in which you find yourself today.

The Habitat Affect 9 Enrichments Experience provides a totally novel way of looking at the all-round inner you and how you can use this information to make lasting changes.

Why enrichment?

To enrich our lives sounds like a noble thing to do – and of course it is. The word 'enrichment' implies improvement, development, progress, moral value and growth – enhancing the chance to experience vitality and happiness.

The ultimate aim is to enrich our lives so that we, in turn – one way or another – enrich the lives of the people with whom we come into contact. Our personal enrichment can also involve little steps to take care of our beautiful planet – the global organ which sustains every single living thing.

A novel way of looking

The 9 Enrichments Experience presented in Part 2 is a special tool which encourages you to assess your current life choices alongside your living spaces. By so doing, you can enhance opportunities for positive achievements and enable your innate happiness to shine through.

The 9 Enrichments cover the many facets of life – work and career; love and romance; life-long learning, respect for parents, seniors and teachers; finance and fortune; health – body and mind; friends, social activity, eco-awareness, travel and adventure; creating and finishing projects, luck of children, celebration; solitude, contemplation and spirituality; confidence, courage and inspiration.

The Magic Square

The template for the 9 Enrichments is a mathematical set known as a Magic Square. Examples of Magic Squares have been found in the artefacts of several early civilizations including those inhabiting the areas we now refer to as Asia and the Middle East. Our 9 Enrichments Magic Square is based on a simple 3 row by 3 column template that is associated with ancient Chinese Feng Shui.

4	9	2
3	5	7
8	1	6

Notice that whichever way you read it – horizontally, vertically, diagonally – the three digits add up to the same number – hence its 'magic' title.

What is the significance of these numbers for my well-being?

Each number has traditionally been associated with 'an enrichment' which represents specific attributes of your psychology, your personality and way of life, and the potential influence of your surrounding habitat.

In our contemporary version, the 9 Enrichments Experience encompasses the breadth of human characteristics and opportunities, but in a way that you are unlikely to have considered before. Perversely, because this is an unfamiliar system for considering how you relate to life's challenges, you are more likely to use it as the means by which you can make an entirely fresh start.

In slightly more detail, here is a summary of the attributes of the 9 Enrichments, each of which comprises human endeavour, a compass direction and one of 5 natural elements – water – earth – wood – metal – fire [also see Appendix L: Compass and element chart].

The 1st Enrichment: work; career; vocation; volunteering; using skills; hidden potential; consolidation of ideas; planning; hibernation; the seed waiting in the ground; north; water.

The 2nd Enrichment: personal relationships; love; romance; sex; compromise; companionship; the joy of sharing; being contently single; finding a soulmate; south west; earth.

The 3rd Enrichment: life-long learning; curiosity; engaging new ideas; personal growth; respect for parents, ancestors, elders, teachers, leaders; germination; initiation; east; wood.

The 4th Enrichment: fortunate blessings; money; prosperity; wealth; planning and budgeting; knowing what is enough for one's needs; generosity; altruism; south east; wood.

The 5th Enrichment: physical health; mental and emotional well-being; harmony; finding a balance; equanimity; patience; honesty and responsibility; the Tai Chi – the centre; earth.

The 6th Enrichment: friendship; guides and helpful people; giving help to others; care for the environment; leisure and social; travel and adventure; appreciation; north west; metal.

The 7th Enrichment: creativity – bringing projects to fruition; nullifying procrastination; harvesting; celebration; relaxation; luck of children; family time; fun; surprises; west; metal.

The 8th Enrichment: sanctuary; humanitarian and spiritual inquiry; belief; faith; reflection; meditation; solitude; meaning; mortality; morality; integrity; thanksgiving; north east; earth.

The 9th Enrichment: self-esteem; action; motivation; confidence; empowerment; fame; expression; inspiration; recognition; significance; experiencing life fully; south; fire.

The 5 Elements represented in Focus Features

As we've noted, each of the 9 Enrichments is associated with a particular compass direction and one of 5 natural elements. The significance of each direction with its associated element is covered in Part 2 where we make specific 'Focus Feature' suggestions for all areas of your home or workplace.

Focus Features are design concepts, décor and placements for you to try using the 5 elements symbolically [see Appendix M – The 5 Elements – for more detail]. These recommended 'makeovers' to your surroundings act as physical 'Habitat Affect' signals in support of your choices-for-change and enrichment experiences.

Compass directions and the sun's energy

At this stage, it is sufficient to remind ourselves that the compass directions relate to the position of the sun vis-a-vis our constantly orbiting planet. All earth's energy ultimately originates from our sun, expressed directionally in a daily and seasonal cycle. It is the sun's energy which ultimately sustains the life force in all living things.

Our personal environmental experience is influenced by our particular situation on the planet in relation to the earth's reception of energy radiating from the sun. There are several variables which affect us to a greater or lesser degree. These include the directional influence of being in the north, the south, the east or the west; whether it's night, dawn, day or dusk; where we're located on the lines of latitude and longitude [our country of residence]; the season – winter, spring, summer or autumn and, of course, the weather!

We can get a sense of this energy influence when we think about how the location of a room or a landscape dramatically affects its 'feel' and often the way 'we feel and think' when we are in that environment. For instance, imagine in your mind's eye how you feel on a cold rainy grey day compared to a bright sunny one.

Getting familiar with your energy environment

Now think for a moment about your own 'energy environment' in and around your home. Can you appreciate the difference between a cool room in the north and a radiant room in the south at mid-day? Can you pick up that fresh feel in the east first thing in the morning? Notice the relaxing energy of the setting sun in the west. With an appreciation of the different 'feel' of the north, the south, the east and the west, you can learn to work with, and enjoy, the available energy.

EAST: initiating energy – new beginnings – growth – morning – spring – fresh light. Feel the fresh awakening of the sunrise and the springtime. Break away from dormant restraints and start something new.

SOUTH: vital energy – expansion – inspiration – mid-day – summer – heat. Feel the vibrant heat and brightness of mid-day and summer. Develop and expand your thoughts and actions on the stage of life.

WEST: transforming energy – fruition – harvesting – afternoon – autumn – mellow warmth. Feel the mellow glowing warmth of late afternoon and autumn. Bring your projects to fruition, celebrate and be thankful for your gifts.

NORTH: stable energy – consolidation – realisation – night – winter – cool reflection. Feel the cool reflective energy of night and winter. Acknowledge your potential, plan for your future; rest and prepare for re-birth.

Outline plan

Although not essential at this stage, if you feel so inclined, you can draw an outline plan of your home [including the surrounding land, if any] with windows, doors and compass directions marked on. This will give you a better feel for the directional energy influencing the various rooms and areas of your property.

Keep your plan as you may want to refer to it as you engage with the 9 Enrichments in Part 2, and also in the final Chapter: 'Sustaining an enriched way of life', where we summarise the Focus Features that are recommended for each direction.

Extra forces of nature

As well as the primal light-heat solar energy – there are other energies prevailing in and around our homes – some healthy, some detrimental. For instance, think of the energy in flowing water – a cleansing shower or a leaking pipe; fresh air from a gentle breeze wafting through an open window or stale putrid air in a damp cold corner; computer and household electrical equipment; artificial lighting; magnetic metals [even found in under-wired bras]; microwaves from ovens and cell phones; the multiplex of sounds – acoustic energy; the heat from a cooker or log burning stove.

Then there's the force of gravity; atmospheric pressure; thunder and lightning; disease in our bodies – infected lethargic energy; polluting energy from inhaling domestic cleaners or eating pesticide residues on our food; our lively household pets; the energy from our own laughter!

Becoming acquainted with all the energy influences in your home is an interesting exercise. Determining which ones are pleasant and helpful, and which ones are damaging or just plain annoying, can help you to create a better atmosphere in which to develop your skills, improve your relationships and celebrate the good things in your life.

Environment-by-design and intuitive Feng Shui

In contemporary western society, people with a thirst for exploring traditions from other cultures, are expressing an interest in Feng Shui. Briefly this is the practice of achieving psychological and physical well-being using environmental design to produce a healthy flow of energy.

The concept of 'the enrichments' comes from oriental Feng Shui practice with its focus on environmental influences and the introduction of measures to 'cure' imperfections and increase supportive elements. In the Habitat Affect, we have adopted the enrichment concept and redeveloped it in a contemporary experiential way as a catalyst for your ability to initiate change and thereby to flourish.

Some of the recommended enrichment actions in Part 2 involve the subtle use of elemental Feng Shui – for instance our Focus Feature suggestions. In this regard, we make no paranormal or spiritual claims about how they actually work. We do, however, acknowledge 'the placebo effect'.

This is a scientifically-recognised beneficial outcome which cannot be attributed to any properties of the treatment itself or, in this case, your Focus Feature activity. The placebo effect has been shown to produce outstanding results in medical research studies. Other psychological phenomena also play a part in the success of your Habitat Affect venture – we mention these influences throughout Part 1.

Does the Habitat Affect differ from other self-help guidance?

Every one of us is a unique human being, we are all different. Rather than 'the one-size-fits-all' approach – simply offering advice and opinions – this book provides you with a novel, easy-to-use system for highly personalised inquiry and exploration. It is a bespoke guide, designed to let you question yourself and discover your own special answers – answers and insights that exactly match your particular circumstances and home environment.

Using a tailor-made approach ensures that the specific choices-for-change you decide to make in your thinking, attitudes, habits, actions and lifestyle, are 'owned by you'. Complementing this, you can undertake the enjoyable physical process of creating harmonious surroundings in your home by following some of our proposals for introducing Focus Features.

Because you find your own highly personalised solutions for the mode of living and surroundings that 'feel right and healthy for you', it is more likely that you will achieve tangible results and lasting benefits.

In this regard, we strongly urge you to use your common sense and follow your intuition, rather than blindly following our recommendations. And, as everyone is different, if you happen to live with other people, there will always be a need to compromise which, in itself, is character-building.

Putting into practice your choices-for-change can also be a fun experience. In a year from now, your life will certainly be more productive and probably a whole lot cheerier.

Your personal choice-creation environment

To re-iterate: the life you experience is the result of an amazing blend of your inherited characteristics, your nurture influences and the choices you make. Family relationships, social and cultural norms, educational opportunity and residential situation – plus a certain amount of luck [however you choose to define it] – all play a part. As the scope of the 9 Enrichments Experience is wide-ranging, it allows you to understand your own mix of needs and aspirations.

Before going into the detail of each specific enrichment and our Habitat Affect suggestions in Part 2, we invite you to reflect on your current home environment in a general way and the 21st century context in which your life plays out.

Over the course of the next few chapters, we explore various factors that influence the choices you make today and hence the life you experience tomorrow. This exploration includes current lifestyle issues, fields of study and common emotional baggage that either help or hinder your choices and well-being. The factors are not mutually exclusive – there is overlap – as with most things in life, interdependence is the pattern.

Lao Tzu, the ancient Chinese sage, said: *"The journey of a thousand miles begins with the first step."*, so let's begin by taking the first step and then another and another ....!

3. SENSUAL CLUTTER-FREE SETTINGS

"The fact is that no species has ever had such wholesale control over everything on earth, living or dead, as we now have. That lays upon us, whether we like it or not, an awesome responsibility. In our hands now lies not only our own future, but that of all other living creatures with whom we share the earth." David Attenborough.

The environments in which we live affect our lives – for better or for worse. This is recognised the world over from the debilitating consequences of living in a manmade slum to the application of certain colours in western hospital settings or the landscaping of community parks. We all live in buildings of one kind or another, surrounded by beauty, mediocrity or even ugliness. With this in mind, it could be your mission to make your daily environmental experience a nourishing affair.

Your personal Habitat Affect relates to the many physical influences of the places you inhabit which can be broadly summarised in four categories.

[1] the enclosed areas within which you live – at home, at work, at play – the specific features of the rooms and open spaces therein. This includes room size and shape: ceiling height – low beams [oppressive bearing down], or too high and out of proportion; square, rectangular or L-shaped rooms – square rooms tend to feel less crowded and cosier than rectangular ones.

Large rooms or long narrow ones can be aesthetically adjusted [eg. a well-positioned attractive screen] to create a more intimate feel and easier positioning of furniture; partitioning in workplace environments to produce discrete personalised territory is deemed to have a biological basis for encouraging productivity.

Other major factors are the position and size of doors and windows with their associated compass directions which dictate the amount of natural sunlight energy; the positioning and use of artificial lighting; fresh air and ventilation.

[2] the building type, external building features, a garden if you have one, and the immediate environment surrounding your home [or workplace], for instance: other buildings, landscape features [topography] and local amenities.

[3] the environments that you use for transport or seek out for relaxation – your car, your train commute, your local park, your leisure club, your chosen walking trails.

[4] the wider global environment where you can play a role, however small. For instance, you can be meticulous about avoiding waste – food, energy, water, transport fuel, surplus clothes – recycling as much as possible.

You can choose to avoid products that contain pollutants or non-essential goods such as products that contain palm oil [which is implicated in the decimation of animal habitats], or make-up/toothpaste that contains plastic micro-beads. You can support educational projects in the developing world and, when possible, try to share your surplus resources for the benefit of others through sponsorship or charitable donations.

Take a look around

Revealingly, what you have chosen to surround yourself with may be indicative of what is going on in your life. This 'surroundings influence' can include the way you interact with others which, in turn, elicits their behaviour towards you. Bearing this in mind, over the next few days you might like to take a look around your home, your garden, your office, your neighbourhood. It can be interesting to discover what sights, sounds, textures, tastes and smells remind you of unpleasantness, conflict or discontent? More importantly, you can explore the sights, sounds, textures, tastes and smells that make you feel good to be alive.

It is quite surprising how many people surround themselves with furniture, objects or pictures, which subconsciously remind them of failed relationships and sad times, or items that are completely irrelevant to their current lives. Others chose to live in poorly illuminated rooms surrounded by ugly clutter or broken items. Then there are those who buy into the latest interior design, irrespective of whether or not it is true to their nature. Some end up living in a home that is more like a show room or hotel. Eccentrics apart, there is little that is nurturing and supportive about any of these environments but, with a little effort, they can easily be improved.

Size is not necessarily an issue

If your home is smaller than you would like and you are feeling hard done by – take heart from the spirited words of Etty Hillesum [1913-1943], a young Jewish woman living in Amsterdam in 1942. When the Nuremburg laws were applied to the Netherlands Etty wrote: *"Take what little space we are left with, fathom its possibilities and use them to the full."*

The smaller your living space, the more creative you may need to be to accommodate your necessities and a few luxuries – yet rising to the challenge can be very rewarding.

Creating a supportive atmosphere

Are you more likely to smile on a sunny day? Do grey clouds and drizzle leave you feeling dull or depressed? Yes, the weather certainly affects most of us. Our subconscious minds 'read' the weather conditions of outdoor environments and we respond accordingly.

In the same way, our indoor environment affects us, from sick building syndrome to that inexplicable uncomfortable feeling we get when a room just isn't quite 'right'. The other side of the coin is a home that is nurturing – one that positively enhances our ability to be or to do whatever we need at the time – to do a good job, to be happy, to be relaxed.

Here we offer a brief guide to the main sensual factors that create your environmental experience – think about your own home or workplace surroundings as you read them.

Visual atmosphere – everything you see influences you to a greater or lesser extent – the colour of the walls, the furniture, the lighting, objects and pictures displayed. Light, which enables our vision, is the primal essence. You can appreciate the balance of visual stimuli by looking at the way harmony is achieved in nature.

Auditory atmosphere – everything you hear influences you. From beautiful music to irritating intrusive noise; from birdsong to barking dogs; from the laughter of children to the sound of running water. Music is used by many organisations to create 'atmosphere' and promote feelings of well-being – a useful tool for shops, encouraging you to relax and buy their goods! Likewise, you can play your favourite tunes at home to arouse you for action or to relax and calm you down.

Tactile atmosphere – everything you can touch and feel influences you. Take a look at the texture of materials, floor coverings, furniture and objects around you. Whether smooth, rough, jagged or volatile, like water as you wash your hands, touch affects us. Medical evidence implies that someone recovering from a heart attack who strokes a pet regularly, may recover quicker with a better future prognosis.

Olfactory atmosphere – everything you smell influences you – from bad odour decay to the wonderful aroma of food and flowers. Big business understands the power of smell – supermarkets use the smell of fresh baked bread to entice us to spend more. Distinct smells can sometimes trigger vivid memories from childhood. You can choose to surround yourself with helpful aromas – smell the roses!

Harmonious atmosphere – based on the duality principle of balancing Yin-Yang elements, you can create a 'feel-good' environment. For example, where there are straight lines introduce some curves, where it is too dark bring in sources of illumination, where it is chilly balance with warmth, and where a room is stale find ways to re-fresh the space.

Psychic atmosphere – are you one of those people who perceives subtle energies associated with certain places or with the people who have previously inhabited them? Do you ever 'feel' that a place is inherently 'good' while another is inherently 'evil'? Some people believe that energy traces from the past persist in ways that currently defy description. However, this doesn't mean that, in the future, an explanation will not be forthcoming. The quantum world is full of surprises.

How does your home or workplace atmosphere measure up?

Is there obvious room for improvement? If so, you will find plenty of suggestions in Part 2 of this book, but by all means make a few adjustments right away – anything that enhances 'the feel-good factor' of a room or area.

Any issues with clutter?

Ask yourself this question: the space I live in is a reflection of myself, does it do me justice? You are invited to decide what is, and what is not, relevant to your life today. Look around you and be ultra-critical for a moment. Have you built up mountains or molehills of papers, clothes, ornaments and accessories over the years? Have you got 'busy' décor and too much furniture? What's hanging on your walls?

Do you believe that 'now' is a good time to simplify your surroundings and your life? If so, you can start to declutter right away using the information below. Alternatively, you can wait till you've read through Part 2 where you will find specific suggestions for cleansing each of the 9 Enrichment areas – you choose the ones that feel right for you. Meanwhile, here are some general clutter-busting actions that really work as a permanent feature of your lifestyle.

The Habitat Affect A-B-C of managing clutter

[A] Arrange attractive practical storage and display areas for absolutely everything that is important and relevant to you;

[B] Recycle, sell, throw out or give away everything that is no longer relevant to your well-being;

[C] Develop an 'easy-for-you' system for everyday 'stuff' and for handling all new incoming items.

Sounds pretty straightforward when put like this – but oh how difficult we make it! So let's be hands-on with some specific practical actions for you to try.

5 clutter-busting solutions that really work in practice

[1] **Does this make my heart sing?** Start by determining what is really 'important and relevant' to you and what is not? Of every item or arrangement in your home, ask yourself the question 'does this make my heart sing'? If your answer is 'no', then it could be hindering you at a subconscious level. Even items necessary for purely functional reasons can have a sense of appeal to them, whether it be a trash can, a saucepan or a towel rail – we all deserve beauty to enrich us every day.

[2] **Where does it live?** Adopt the standard that 'everything in my home has a home of its own'. So every single item has a specific place for storage or display when not in active use. Anything without 'a recognised home' in your home, garden or office, that you need to keep should be given suitable storage right away. Thereafter everything else can be treated in one of the following 6 ways:

- sell the item;
- recycle or freecycle the item;
- gift it to a friend or family member;
- loan it to a friend or family member;
- donate it to charity with gift aid;
- throw it away as trash.

Be strong and ruthless in your determination to distinguish between what is worth keeping and what needs to leave your life for good.

[3] **First take everything out.** When starting to tackle an untidy cluttered area – a room or desk, cupboard or drawer, or wherever your clutter congregates – the rule is 'first take everything out' [apart from heavy

furniture – although you may want to remove some of this permanently!]. Now replace each item one by one asking 'does this make my heart sing'? If the answer is 'no' then sell, recycle, give away or throw it out. If the item is something functional that you really need, but it doesn't make your heart sing, then think about ways of beautifying it or, if you can afford to do so, buy a replacement.

[4] **Dealing with computer storage.** Use the same logic when dealing with computer files and folders. Are they chaotic and disorganised or do you have an easy-to-use system for storage and retrieval? What about your back-up systems – external hard drive, USB sticks, cloud storage? Are there thousands of e-mails lingering in your mail boxes? Is your desktop full of icons? What about your smart phone – all those Apps you never use? Set aside a dedicated clean-up day once a quarter and ensure your systems work effectively for your particular e-lifestyle.

[5] **Challenging psychological issues.** Some of us hold onto 'stuff' for years out of habit without understanding why? If there are deeper psychological issues for you to challenge, you might consider attending a clutter-busting workshop or do a spot of self-detective work – ask yourself why 'such and such' is important to you today? Sometimes making connections with the past can be difficult, so go easy on yourself. The sheer exhilaration of being in a clutter-free environment surrounded by things that 'make your heart sing' will be well worth the effort.

The designer, artist and writer William Morris is famously quoted as saying: *"Have nothing in your house that you do not know to be useful, or believe to be beautiful."* This maxim perfectly summarises the technique for creating an enriching environment which is what this book is all about.

4. THE POWER OF COLOUR AND PLANTS IN YOUR HABITAT

"Those who are awake, live in a state of constant amazement." Buddha. Our world is full of colour and also full of plants which use colour in the most wonderful ways. If you open your eyes wide to these glorious gifts of nature, you can experience a tremendous sense of wonder for the beauty of the spectacle.

Colour in our lives

The colours in our surroundings can affect us deeply. Just imagine a world without colour. Colour can be uplifting, yet colour can also issue warning signals, dangers to be avoided. Colour can deceive. Environments which lack colour can be drab and depressing – viz 'the grey day'. At its best, colour can be calming or invigorating, colour can refresh and inspire us. Colour can be a feast for the eyes and a tonic for the mind.

In a thought-provoking interview with architect Will Alsop concerning 'Colour in Architecture', he says: "Not only does colour influence the way in which we experience a structure, its intelligent use also helps to express the building's identity and enhances its users' involvement.

"How we see things also depends on the time of day as sunlight moves from a blue tinge to a yellowish one. But our brains have adjusted to take account of this so we see a red flower being the same red in the morning as the evening – we call this colour constancy."

The amazing spectrum of light energy

Colours are a form of light energy [photons] transmitted in different wavelengths from infrared to ultraviolet with all the hues of red, orange, yellow, green, blue and indigo in between – think of a radiant rainbow.

Low frequency infrared is low energy light and high frequency ultra violet is high energy light. High energy ultra violet [UV ray] is well known to sun bathers as potentially dangerous light. On the other hand, birds of prey use it for stalking their quarry – their victim's urine leaves a trail which is visible courtesy of the bird-eye UV receptors. The term 'eagle eyes' is well founded.

Complementary colours

White contains all colour potentialities. Black is the absence of colour. Red, blue and yellow are the three primary pigments. Complementary colours are colours opposite each other on 'the colour wheel' – a way of representing the entire colour spectrum in circular format which, if spun rapidly, appears white.

Knowing which colours complement each other is useful for interior design purposes. Red complements green [yellow + blue]; yellow complements violet [red + blue]; blue complements orange [red + yellow].

Appendix A provides descriptions of common colours and their attributes to help you make interior design choices that can have a positive influence on your experiences.

Introducing appropriate colours as Focus Features

In Part 2 of the Habitat Affect you will find various Focus Feature recommendations based on suitable colours for particular areas of your home. For now, have a think about colour as it presently features in your life. Which colours are your own particular favourites? What is it about them that you like? How do you use them in your surroundings, your clothes, the foods you eat? What does your choice of colours tell you about yourself? Appendix A, as already mentioned, may help you to think more about the colours in your life.

Living with plants

As human beings we owe our lives to the plant kingdom because they are natural manufacturers of carbohydrates. It is their ability to capture the sun's cosmic energy through a process known as photosynthesis that gives us food for nourishment and our life-sustaining atmosphere.

Photosynthesis takes place within the leaves of green plants during sunlit hours in the presence of the catalyst chlorophyll [which is responsible for the green colour]. This amazing process converts carbon dioxide and water molecules into energy-rich carbohydrate molecules.

These carbohydrates form the basis of our food chain, providing vital calories [energy] that we need for a healthy diet. We obtain the calories either directly when we eat plant material or indirectly when we consume animals that have eaten plants – herbivores – or animals who themselves have eaten other animals – carnivores.

Oxygen – essential for our existence

Most foods [fungi being an exception] can be traced back to the process of photosynthesis. But that's not all – the by-product of photosynthesis is oxygen – the gas we personally rely on for our very being. This is why safeguarding the world's rainforests as valuable capital assets, is crucial to the well-being of our planet. It is vitally important to encourage those nations with large forested areas, possibly with financial incentives, to halt the desecration of their tree-scapes.

On a more modest scale, aside from nutrition and healthy air, the plants or even pictures of plants in our living rooms, gardens and workplaces can influence us beneficially in several ways which are important if you are aiming to create a healthy Habitat Affect.

Vital plant power

Plants are sensual – they inspire us visually and aromatically. Their predominant 'green' is the colour in the middle of the rainbow representing balance and healing. Flowers come in a fantastic array of colours and fragrances and have all sorts of associations. Choose the ones that make you feel good.

According to Feng Shui tradition, plants are said to move vital 'life force' energy – Chi – around. Broad leaved plants can encourage the flow of good Chi, while spiky plants may introduce the 'poison arrows' of bad 'cutting Chi', so you are advised to be careful where you position them.

Broad leaved plants are used as a remedy to help block any 'poison arrows' which are, allegedly, emitted via jutting pointed objects, sharp jagged edges, the proud corner of an L shaped room, the inauspicious position of surrounding buildings, straight roads aiming directly at your front door or long narrow corridors.

However, rather than sticking rigidly to the prescriptive rules of others, your own cultural norms and preferences are by far the best guide. For instance, the Yucca plant is spiky and yet, if you live in Peru, it is essential to the agricultural landscape where it forms protective hedging. In UK tradition, displaying red-berried Holly in December acts as a convivial decoration; in the US, Poinsettia is a seasonal favourite.

Anti-pollutant and uplifting properties

Over the last 20 years or so, the proliferation of home and workplace electronic equipment has been immense. Today many of us are living and working in highly charged indoor environments. Interestingly NASA has shown that plants can absorb excess harmful electro-magnetic pollution. To benefit from this purging effect, it is recommended that there should be at least one broad leaved plant by every computer in an office. Similarly, if you have a fixed computing area at home, placing a potted plant nearby is a good idea.

If you want to instantly enliven a room, fresh flowers in a vase will do the trick; likewise gazing out of a picture window at colourful garden flowers is a distinctly uplifting experience.

"If we could see the miracle of a single flower clearly, our whole life would change." Buddha.

5. YOUR LIFE IN THE ROUND

"So often time it happens, we all live our life in chains, and we never even know we have the key." The Eagles [Already Gone]. In this chapter we delve into some key issues which may impact your life and your use of the Habitat Affect.

To begin with, let's consider just how dramatically western civilisation has changed over the last half century. Even allowing for the global recession, many of us have enough, and more, to fulfil our every basic need – yet we may feel there is still something missing.

As developed societies have generally become more affluent, the number of people seeking help for anxiety, depression and stress-related problems has risen at an alarming rate – some estimates say by as much as 300% in the UK since the 1950s. The dramatic rise in prescription drugs for stress-related conditions and depression is well documented. Insecurity and isolation are on the increase. Even as we bask in plenty, some of us still feel miserable – why is this? How can we create 'a climate of blue sky consent' rather than 'a climate of grey sky dissent' when we come to make the choices and decisions that affect the quality of our daily lives?

Under pressure? How about some self-discipled willpower?

What are the pressures that are seemingly infecting our lives? Is it our ultra-competitive workplaces? Bad news about jobs and the economy? Sex and violence overload in the media? Family breakdown? Unsatisfying personal relationships? Poor nutrition? Lack of exercise? Low self-esteem? Alcohol or drug abuse? Gambling? Anxiety over sexual performance? Fear of failure? Fear of ageing? Fear of terrorism? Religious intolerance? Financial worry and debt? Lack of educational opportunity? No sense of belonging to a cohesive local community? Being in a spiritual desert? The grip of materialistic shopping? Internet and digital overload? An unnatural need for constant auditory or visual stimulation? Compulsive searching for pleasurable distractions? A need for instant gratification? Helplessness because others seem to have all the power and control? Vacuous celebrity culture? A lack of positive role models with a moral compass?

These pressures sound pretty overwhelming when listed together but fortunately you are unlikely to meet them all during your lifetime, although you will almost certainly be conflicted by one or more of these challenges. However, for every unhelpful pressure that you do experience or are exposed to, rather than succumb, there is always an alternative way to think and to behave.

The alternative requires that, however difficult, you harness your willpower. You identify pressures that have personal impact and learn to change your approach. From among the vast variety of inducements on offer, you purposely develop active discrimination. You 'mind-train' yourself, over a period of time, to substitute helpful thoughts and actions.

Being conscientious about taking personal responsibility for your choices, and having the courage to meet your demons head-on, will allow you to make the most of the many opportunities that life has to offer.

Are you living up to your potential?

We are born and we die, that much is certain. Between these two events, we live in a constantly changing uncertain world. We have been gifted this amazing opportunity to experience life. We have the potential either to squander this gift or to engage it in a purposeful way to the benefit of all. So the question is: "am I living up to my potential?".

Every one of us is an incredible mix of inherited traits, learned responses and ingrained habits, fixed and flexible beliefs, creativity and, above all, we are conscious beings. Consciousness is defined as the state of being aware of, and responsive to, one's surroundings.

How we experience the world depends on our conscious mindset – our awareness of the potential we have to flourish or to suffer within our surroundings. Take the spectrum of emotional experiences, ranging from destructive fear, anger, resentment, guilt, jealousy, despair and sadness to constructive kindness, compassion, courage, altruism, joy, love and bliss. We all have the capacity to engage this variety of emotions.

Why spend this precious lifetime 'suffering' in a destructive mindset when you have the potential for a dynamic, loving, compassionate identity – a way of being that is so much more fulfilling? But for all sorts of reasons, this is what many of us do, at least some of the time. In order to optimise the potential for health, happiness and a purposeful life, it is necessary to escape from 'destructive' influences and adopt a 'constructive' mindset.

Can you accept 'what is' and find the silver lining?

As we become positively constructive in our way of thinking, so we develop a mindset that accepts 'what is'. In particular, we learn to acknowledge and accept changed circumstances following difficult or disturbing episodes in our lives.

Acceptance of 'what is' includes the opportunity to find insight in hardship, to learn valuable lessons and ultimately to gain from experience. In this regard, you can use your personally-devised Habitat Affect to reinforce a constructive approach, particularly during the inevitable times of difficulty.

Nearly every cloud really can have a silver lining – the obese person becomes the inspiring slimming club leader, the drug addict becomes the role model for how to quit, the death of a loved one from a tragic accident or evil deed results in a charity that helps others in a similar position.

There are numerous examples of heroes and heroines who have come to accept that the past cannot be changed but the future can be radically different. The secret is always – repeat always – to accept 'what is', look for 'the silver lining' and use its lesson as a guidepost for the present and the future.

How do you feel about uncertainty and change?

Out there in 'the real world' uncertainty reigns supreme – change happens – everything in the universe is in a constant state of flux. And our lives are no exception. Contrarily, although impossible, there is an enduring human desire for certainty and permanence. The very familiarity of the status quo, however difficult, often seems easier to live with than taking a leap into the void of the uncertain unknown.

Some changes can be anticipated such as age-related deterioration which is balanced by the wisdom of mature experience. However most lives are touched by completely unexpected changes that happen 'out of the blue'. While some of these can be good news, others may be extremely hurtful and tragic. The latter can instantaneously result in a state of shock which may well require medical intervention. Herein we are focusing on less damaging changes, but changes nonetheless which could have a significant impact on your future health and happiness.

Do you expect the unexpected?

If an uninitiated change occurs, it is often viewed as a complete surprise when, in fact, we should all be primed to 'expect the unexpected'. When taken off guard, we tend to 're-act' anxiously to the unforeseen circumstances and these reactions may not always be the most appropriate course for our well-being.

Therefore a key ingredient for a happy life is to adopt an outlook that expects and embraces change and uncertainty. Over time you can learn to work with uncertainty and even learn to benefit from its challenges, however uncomfortable or distressing your circumstances may initially appear. In so doing, you can think and act more calmly and appropriately when taken by surprise.

Better still, you can go along with uncertainty and choose to create your own change. This is the best means of enriching the way you live. Whether it is your eating habits, taking time to make a grandparent laugh or deciding on a new career path, you are in the driving seat. You are the only person who intuitively knows the answer to the question "what changes do I need to make so that I can embrace uncertainty and still manage to have a good life?".

How well do you cope with life's ups and downs?

The most difficult periods can be the times of greatest gain – the times when you develop inner strength, resilience and appreciation for those who have supported you.

Plato gave us words of wisdom which are as true today as they were in 400 BC. *"How singular is the thing called pleasure, and how curiously related to pain, which might be thought to be the opposite of it, for they never come to a person together. And yet, those who pursue either of them are generally compelled to take the other. They are two, and yet they grow together out of one head or stem."*

This suggests that pleasure and pain are two sides of the same coin. If we pursue one, we open ourselves up to experience the other. Yet even within painful experience there can be a constructive aspect, for it is in learning from our weaknesses and our pain, as well as from our strengths and our pleasures, that we make real progress.

When everything is going brilliantly, it is easy to be happy, and that we can celebrate. The extra challenge is to maintain a life well-lived when times are hard and difficulties encircle us. After all, if self-improvement and feeling purposeful were an instant quick-fix, then we would all have it sorted by now.

The philosopher Epictetus [AD 55-135] suggested that it is not events themselves that cause us to have problems, but rather our beliefs and opinions about those events. You alone have the power to view your daily dramas, problems and suffering as opportunities for learning, change and renewal. On this note the Chinese word for 'crisis' is made up of two components, the symbol for 'danger' and the symbol for 'opportunity'. Each time you experience the painful side of life, you can also explore the inherent opportunity.

Are your fears, doubts and worries hindering you?

In the famous words of Franklin D Roosevelt: *"The only thing we have to fear is fear itself"*. Many 'apparent' difficulties – the things that ultimately hinder us from leading the sort of lives we would really like – often have their roots in irrational beliefs that give rise to unnecessary fears, doubts and worry. These potentially damaging dreads are not always entirely obvious on the surface.

Hindering fear, debilitating doubt and unnecessary worry can manifest in all sorts of ways from anger to resentment and victim-hood, from procrastination to overwork, from guilt to trying too hard to please, from crippling shyness to talking too much, from self-sabotage to overcompensating behaviour, from worry to yet more worry.

Often you will find, when you think deeply, that your festering fears, doubts and worries are not grounded in fact. Therefore, you are actually allowing yourself to be emotionally or physically afraid of an idea or an imaginary situation. Once recognised and tackled head on, your fears and doubts can cease to be a massive barrier to accomplishing whatever it is that you would truly love to be or to do.

According to Shakespeare in Measure for Measure: *"Our doubts are traitors, and make us lose the good we oft might win by fearing to attempt."*

If you want to examine your fears and worries in more detail, including specific action suggestions, please see Appendix B where we cover this subject in some detail. Please note: if you are in actual danger of being physically or mentally abused, then your fears are well founded and you should seek professional assistance.

Have you thought about simplifying the way you live?

Would you say that your life always flows along with 'the natural order' of things? Unlikely, unless you happen to live in an unspoilt habitat so far undiscovered by 21st century humankind!

However, there are many things we can all do to live more naturally and simply, at the same time helping to cut down planetary pollution and increase the chances of having a healthy life. Starting from the basis that the natural order is one of interdependence – everything affects everything else – you might take an objective look at your current lifestyle.

You may decide to do some research into food options for eating more unprocessed plant-based meals, taking regular good quality exercise [walking is free], cutting down on wasteful habits, recycling clothes and household goods, and prioritising what is truly important to you and your loved ones.

Naturally if you have children, their needs take precedence over yours. Earning a viable living and giving them as much of your time and attention as is appropriate for their mental and physical welfare, must be an absolute priority.

If you do choose to live more simply, you will find the added benefit is that you have fewer possessions to worry about. Nearly 2000 years ago Epictetus gave us a brilliant piece of advice: *"If you want to develop your ability to live simply, do it for yourself, do it quietly, and don't do it to impress others."*

6. UNDERSTANDING YOUR CHOICES

"Destiny is not a matter of chance, it is a matter of choice." William Jennings Bryan. When you entertain thoughts or behave in a certain way, are you always aware that this is a matter of your choosing? What about your current home environment – the décor, furniture, objects and images which you have chosen as your surroundings – the qualities that comprise your personal Habitat Affect?

The future you get depends on causes and conditions – many of which are a direct result of the conscious choices and decisions that you make on a daily basis. However, your choices are often influenced on a subtle level by a range of subliminal phenomena including priming and nudging, the way a question is framed, previous experience and exposure, even karma.

Some neuroscientists and philosophers claim that 'free will' to choose is an illusion – the debate continues. However, for the purposes of developing your personal Habitat Affect, it is useful to explore what may be going on consciously and subconsciously behind your decision-making.

Choosing choice

In order to make good choices for your future benefit, you actively have to choose what to choose. This may sound obvious yet we believe it warrants discussion. Making a choice is a proactive effort, otherwise life would just 'happen' to you – happy or sad – when your 'say in the matter' is limited or even non-existent. How much more sensible it is to bring your conscience considerate mind to bear on your daily decisions.

This means you alone are fundamentally responsible for each 'chosen choice', the outcome of which, you hope, will have the intended consequence you desire. However in life, there are often unintended consequences, so there is a need to be aware of this possibility. Indeed, if an unintended consequence arises, it may involve you in yet more choices.

Unintended consequences

One well-known example of an unintended consequence is the development of the atomic bomb which was 'sold' to the physicists working on it as the best choice of weapon to bring an early end to World War II. On this basis, they chose to work on the bomb at Los Alamos. Today we all live with the unintended consequences – a world full of nuclear weapons. Although some people regard them as 'peace-keeping deterrents', if ever they were deployed, the decimation of our atmosphere and biological ecosystems, including human beings in vast numbers, is certain.

Your particular unintended consequences will be on a different scale, yet for you, they may be of great concern, so always make allowances for unforeseen happenings. It is sensible to 'expect the unexpected' and, however difficult, wise to adopt the practice of being unattached to outcomes.

Priming – framing – nudging

Understanding that you can control many of your choices is quite liberating, especially when there are difficult decisions to be made. However in order to 'own your choices', you need to recognise the context in which they are being made. Research in behavioural economics has demonstrated that people are influenced to a great extent by the way that choices are presented to them – 'priming' and 'framing' – so you need to be aware of this.

For instance, your decisions could be 'primed' by things you see, hear or read in the media. Your choice of media often reinforces views you already hold. Such media information may be a one-sided view – or even an erroneous 'fake news' account – of a particular situation. Fake news is currently a massive issue with the proliferation of social media where anyone can post their version of events – who or what do you choose to believe?

Another case in point is being given a choice between two things when neither is necessarily right for you; advertisers and politicians are good at using this framing tactic. Or you may be primed and framed, by accepting a cup of coffee, to listen to a salesperson you might not otherwise bother with. How about if you attend a function with lots of 'interesting people' and are then coerced into pledging support for 'a good cause' – their cause? Debatably indoctrination is an extreme and highly dangerous form of priming.

Behavioural experts also suggest that people make better choices when they are given 'nudges' – subtle persuaders and sometimes rewards – rather than being forced by legislation. You can think of the Habitat Affect ideas and 9 Enrichments Experience suggestions as being your nudge to make small changes in support of wise choices so you can improve your outcomes and build a healthier lifestyle.

Too much choice

In his iconic 1970 book 'Future Shock', Alvin Toffler predicted: *"People of the future may suffer not from an absence of choice but from a paralysing surfeit of it. They may turn out to be victims of that peculiarly super-industrial dilemma – overchoice."*

Various psychological experiments since then have clearly demonstrated the problem of having too much choice. For instance, subjects find it much harder to make purchasing decisions if presented with too many options. Just think about the massive choice of different varieties of the same type of product in our superstores or the TV and new media channels vying for our attention.

Besides the difficulty of making a simple decision, too much choice can actually be quite stressful. Take the example of contemporary e-devices; it is easy to become overwhelmed by the mass of technical gismos and upgrades, with new ones coming on stream almost weekly – know the feeling? Faced with so many choices, it is difficult to discriminate between all the various communication and viewing options, which incidentally are extremely addictive.

Screen time and content choice

For those of us responsible for children and young adults, there is concern about what constitutes a healthy amount of screen time and appropriate online content. The gamut of subject matter vying for attention is vast: school and college study, coding and entrepreneurial app development, social networking and video topics, violent films, pornographic material, addictive games and virtual relationships. Choices need to be made by all of us – young and old alike – but where to draw the line? Too much interface with modern technology can fuel anxiety, induce physical tension, trigger poor posture and obviously restrict the amount of time available for other, possibly healthier, pursuits.

Academic studies have found that walking briskly on a regular basis, preferably in natural surroundings, can affect brain function in ways that protect memory and thinking skills, lower your blood pressure, strengthen your heart and boost the immune system. This is a simple choice we can all make daily and leave the techno-gismos behind for half an hour. In addition, how about having an 'off-grid' day or two? The idea of taking a tech-free holiday is gaining popularity.

Addressing the key question

A salutary wake-up call to abandon unhelpful habits and make helpful choices is the well-known maxim: *"if you keep on doing what you've always done, you'll keep on getting what you've always got"*. Coupled with this: *"what you sow you will ultimately reap"* begs the ubiquitous 'sixty four thousand dollar' question: "what do I really want?". In other words: "what do I choose to sow – to be, to do, to happen?".

Ironically it is easier to say what you don't want to be, to do or to happen, and much harder to be clear about exactly what it is that you do want. Certain philosophers equate 'freedom' – something we all value – with being able to choose what we want in life. So, given the freedom to make that choice, here are a couple of suggestions.

First try writing a quick list of up to 6 things that you don't want or don't like. Many of us spend hours talking and thinking about the negatives in life, "I don't want so and so", "I don't like such and such", "I don't know how to do ………", "I hate the thought of ………", "I never want to try that again" etc. Notice how easy it is to be negative.

Secondly, try to be both specific and realistic by writing down up to 6 things that you are passionate about and would welcome more of in your life. If you already know some of the choices and changes you might need to make in order to increase the abundance of these things, you can add a few notes and refer back to your list from time to time.

However, at this stage, you are may still be unsure about what you need 'to sow' for a fulfilling future. You can use

43

the 9 Enrichments Experience in Part 2 to clarify your thoughts and aspirations, and then organise your home environment to attract whatever you feel will support your endeavours.

In the 9th Enrichment Experience Action Area, ACTION C is an exercise called 'Fast forward 10 years to view your achievements'. This allows you to explore what you really want to accomplish over the next ten years so you can make the necessary choices to get you there. You may like to engage with it now and then again when you have discovered all the enrichment qualities you want to own.

Did you choose your current habits?

"The difficulty lies not in the new ideas, but in escaping from the old ones." John Maynard Keynes. Previous experience and exposure to an idea or an action can result in habits – either in attitude [prejudice being a negative example] and other emotional responses or in physical actions such as over-eating or too much screen time – the sort of habits you may subconsciously display on a daily basis.

According to research by psychologists, it takes at least 21 days to break an ingrained behavioural habit – 'the clutter habit' for instance, or the habit of diving into the biscuit tin without a moment's thought, the habit of saying 'yes' to keep everybody happy, the habit of negative mental chatter, the habit of being late etc. Can you think of any unhelpful habits you'd like to be rid of?

Knowing about this 3 week habit-breaking period can help you make allowances for the occasional relapse while you are taking part in the 9 Enrichments Experience. Please note we are not talking here about substance addiction such as serious nicotine, alcohol or pain-killer habits which may take substantially longer.

If you do decide to have a go at tackling a habit that you now realise is not useful to your progress, consider that actually three weeks is not that long when you put it into the context of your entire lifetime. It is important to go easy on yourself if you backslide occasionally and have a wry smile when you find that you are still acting in a habitual way which no longer serves you. Seeing the humorous side of quirky habits often helps you to break them and move on.

Being practical 'on purpose' with personal pep-talks

A practical way to break a habit is to 'choose on purpose' to try something specific that is different and find the courage to stick with it even if, to start with, the new something is just a distraction. When you come to make this habit-breaking decision, it is worth taking time to brainstorm all foreseeable outcomes, preferably write them down and think them through.

Although life seldom gives us exactly what we plan for, being awake to possible outcomes can be enormously helpful, provided our expectations are realistic. In fact it is better to get rid of expectations altogether once you have set your course of action.

If you think of your action or non-action as an experiment, then there's no need to expect a right or a wrong outcome, you just get 'a result'. When a particular 'result' is helpful to you, it can become your new habit. If you want to make and reinforce new habits, you can use the Habitat Affect Focus Features [detailed in Part 2] to act as habit-change reminders around you home.

We also recommend uplifting personal pep-talks. Talk to yourself – out loud if necessary – in an enthusiastic manner, telling yourself you have both the courage and determination to stick with a new way of thinking and acting till it becomes second-nature – a habit that serves your life's purpose.

Karma

The Sanskrit word 'karma' means 'action'. Karma is a creative principle, it is what you choose, not what happens to you. The modern misuse of the word tends to imply something that is done to you – "oh it's my bad karma!". When bad things do inevitably happen, you may be able to trace back to some point in the past when there was a poor choice or action. This poor choice may even be of your own making. Realising this, without self-pity or blame because 'what is done, is done', you can choose to see it as a potential learning experience and set the intention of making better choices from now on.

Sometimes individuals appear to suffer 'bad karma' but this is as a result of the decisions and activities of other people, organisations, governments or hazardous inventions that populate the modern world, for example – transport vehicles with the potential to crash and cause injury or even death.

Other ghastly instances of collective bad karma are the case of babies born into abject poverty or civilians living in the middle of a war zone. No-one would expect them to have chosen this situation – the karma of these examples results from the poor choices and actions of others, sometimes way back in history.

You can choose to be an active participant by creating 'good karma' all around you – both by fashioning a supportive home base environment and by the way you interact with the people and places in your life.

Wise decision-making

In order to be true to yourself, you may have to go outside convention when making wise choices as George Bernard Shaw remarked: *"the power of accurate observation is commonly called cynicism by those who have not got it."* When making a choice, accurately observing your various options with the eye of a cynic, may prove to be an important deciding factor.

So, provided you do no harm to others, choose your own life journey as you would like it to be, rather than the life that you think is expected of you by other people and society.

Here's a great saying: *"responsible choices are never unplanned careless reactions."* When faced with a major decision, you may find the 6 Perfections of Buddhist tradition useful as qualities to help you choose wisely. They are: generosity, moral discipline, patience, joyous exertion, contemplation and wisdom. Choices made with these qualities in mind are likely to be responsible ones, creating a purposeful outcome.

Assumptions versus facts

If you would like to delve further into the complex realm of human decision-making, then the work of Nobel Laureate Daniel Kahneman is extremely challenging and helpful. In particular, his book 'Thinking fast and slow' demonstrates how the mind tends to re-act based on assumptions rather than factual information.

Research in the field of behavioural economics and the psychology of decision-making is currently very active. The results may have huge implications for government policy, as well as for private individuals. We are only just beginning to understand how irrational many of our seemingly rational preferences and selections really are.

Even though we may not realise it, we all make daily assumptions – partial judgments – that colour our choices and decisions.

Whatever your set of personal values, every active choice that you make creates your future. With this in mind, you can unleash your personal power to identify and challenge your assumptions, assess the facts as best you can, and thereafter make conscientious choices 'on purpose'. You will be rewarded with experiences that are as enriched as you choose to make them.

"The strongest principle of growth lies in human choice."
George Eliot [Mary Ann Evans].

7. HEALTH AND YOUR BODY

"It is health that is real wealth and not pieces of gold and silver." Mahatma Gandhi.

With an understanding of your capability to choose wisely, you can make positive decisions about how you treat your body. The exciting news from neuroscience is that physical exercise and a healthy diet, along with the right amount of sleep [for you], will help improve your emotional status.

There follows a simplistic summary of health-related topics, while later on in Part 2: the 5th Enrichment Experience, you will be able to explore your personal health issues in some detail and how you can maximise the Habitat Affect to safeguard your physical and mental welfare.

Starting from the premise that everything about you is interdependent, you can begin to appreciate the relationship between the physical aspects of your body, the influence of stimuli in your environment and the biochemistry of your brain which underlies your thoughts and feelings.

Fight or flight

The Habitat Affect relates to the influence of subtle sensations in your surroundings. When you encounter a stimulus of some kind via your five senses [sight, sound, touch, smell, taste] or through a thought arising, the part of your brain that processes the emotions associated with that stimulus [the amygdala] is activated. This emotional centre activation occurs before your reasoning 'cognitive' faculty [the prefrontal cortex] kicks in.

This explains the instant 'fight or flight' reaction. You are doubtless familiar with the adrenaline rush – heart pounding, palms sweating, hairs standing on end – when faced with a fear-provoking situation such as a near miss in dangerous traffic, confronting a snake or a large growling dog, unexpected traumatic news. You simply do not have time to think about it, but you certainly have an immediate physiological and emotional fear reaction in your body.

The fact that the amygdala precedes the prefrontal cortex in processing neural information with an emotional component [many of your thoughts!] also accounts for why it is so difficult to modify behaviour and habits by thinking and reasoning alone. This is the case even when you really want to make some changes.

You may reason that you are going to do, or not do, something and then find that you unwittingly sabotage yourself. Examples of this 'compulsive' behaviour include over-eating, under-eating, obsessing about an ex-partner, sex that plays along with poor self-esteem, drinking too much to numb your mind or relying on prescription or other drugs. Once alcohol or drugs have become a habit, the body's biochemical addiction to the substance itself also has to be dealt with. So it is not just mental reasoning alone that shapes your behaviour and your ability to change.

Let's get physical

It appears that several physical factors – which happily you can do something about – have quite an impact on your brain cells, including the ones in the amygdala. What you do, or don't do, physically helps create the biochemical and bioelectrical condition of your brain and likewise the status of the nerve pathways and heart ganglia – the body's neural substations. In other words, physical activity impacts your mental and emotional well-being, so it is imperative to make healthy physical choices.

Factors such as sedentary lifestyles and poor diets are known to contribute to heart conditions, strokes and Type 2 diabetes – all major health issues today. However, their impact on emotional health is only just beginning to be recognised.

It is vitally important to have an exercise regime that works for you and is pleasant, rather than a chore. It is entirely your choice what form of exercise you take – but we emphasise the essential need for exercise as part of your participation in the 9 Enrichments Experience.

In this respect, putting the Habitat Affect into practice can help to make your exercise routine hassle-free. You could organise an area in your home so that your kit – be it walking boots, running shoes, gym equipment, bicycle, rackets, balls etc – is easy to access. Some people find it helpful to introduce a system whereby they make 'prompting notes' in the diary or on screen of their planned exercise.

When you chose to put some form of daily physical activity on the agenda, you will keep your body functioning well and notice the change in your general well-being remarkably soon. Arranging to do physical activities with other people [friends or join a club] is another useful way to keep on track and you will benefit from the sociability aspect of exercising as a couple or in a group.

Nutritious food and fresh air

There is no avoiding food, we have to eat to live, yet our relationship with food is a complex one. When it comes to eating and drinking, if you are so minded, you can take control of everything you put in your mouth. After all, nobody else is in control of this aspect of your life.

'Yes' you can empower yourself to choose a healthy diet including whole grains, fruits, vegetables, nuts, seeds and foods rich in omega 3 fatty acids 'food for the brain' – the

5th Enrichment Experience goes into detail – and make this way of eating a luxurious habit.

You can also expose yourself to a certain amount of daylight [NB avoid damaging sunbathing] and thereby ensure your Vitamin D levels are optimal. Walking outdoors, preferably in the fresh air with some skin exposed, is highly recommended apart from times of intense sunshine when there is a risk of sunburn. You can also practice 'walking meditation' and breathing exercises in the fresh air.

A good night's sleep

While everybody knows that good quality sleep is essential for well-being, getting the right amount can be problematic for some people. Parents of young babies will be able to tell you all about the downsides of interrupted sleep, indeed sleep deprivation it is a well-recognised form of torture. Yet in today's wired-up 24/7 world many of us are denying ourselves decent sleep by overstimulating our brains just when they should be winding down. Do you recognise this trend in your own life?

Self-discipline around sleep is vitally important. You can choose to arrange your schedule, your surroundings and the time of your last meal to ensure that you get enough quality sleep. If you share a double bed with your partner, you need to respect each other's sleep patterns and possibly use ear plugs, eye shades, two duvets or whatever enables refreshing rest. Resorting to sleeping pills is never a good idea, so always try other options first.

Everything is interconnected

At the quantum physics level, we are all made of constantly moving elementary particles. Your apparent independent existence, and that of all the living beings and things that you see as separate discrete objects in the world, is simply an illusion.

This deceptive impression of reality is fed by human consciousness – the ability to conceptualise on the basis of sensing things as being separate, to label these separate objects or ideas using words which are open to interpretation, and to make observations relative to a particular time and place. Appendix C: Inside the elements describes the perpetual motion of energy at the quantum scale and the elements from which we are all made.

Environmental scientists highlight the synergy of everything and everybody in the universe. On a personal level, this means every part of your life is interconnected and can affect everything you are and do. A simplistic example is the unwelcome interference of minor sickness. When you are ill, it can be very difficult to give your usual full attention to work or whatever activity you are engaged in. With today's unhealthy diets, sedentary lifestyles, frenetic workplaces, lack of sleep, traffic jams and packed trains, many people, while not 'ill', are definitely functioning below par.

On a sensory level, if you hear the sound of running water, your bladder muscles may require more control. In similar vein, if you are exposed to stressful stimuli such as violent images and harsh sounds – brutal computer games, aggressive movies, impoverished street life, dysfunctional relationships – these are going to affect the biochemistry of your body which, in turn, may affect your immune system and your general well-being.

Wholesome healing opportunities

The scientific field of Psycho-Neuro-Immunology [PNI] investigates the impact that sensory and social interactions have on our physical and mental health. It aims to discover the communicating links between the nervous system [our mind processes], the endocrine system [our hormones] and the immune system [our defences for recognising and fighting harmful bacteria, viruses and our own cancer cells].

Ultimately the body – your body – has to heal itself, even when there has been significant help from conventional medicines and possibly surgery. By adopting a way of life that integrates the health of your mind and body, your self-healing mechanisms will have a much better chance of working effectively. With an appreciation of how everything interconnects, there is a desire to live more wholesomely which, in turn, provides opportunities for long-term healing.

Our physical environments provide constant stimulation, via our sense organs, which can be damaging, neutral or nurturing. Similarly, our mental 'cognitive environment' can be harmful or helpful. Perceptions, thoughts, memory, reasoning, emotions, vivid dreams, actions and reactions are inseparable – we are holistic creatures. So when it comes to healing – mental and physical – popular allopathic 'treat the symptom' approaches are not the whole answer.

Even as recently as ten years ago, practical 'whole person' systems for healing and helping people to achieve a vigorous life were rare. Presenting symptoms were [and often still are] treated in isolation with prescription drugs, without taking into account a person's overall physical and emotional condition, and general lifestyle.

Medicalised problems and treatments

While lifestyle is at long last being acknowledged as a contributing factor, we still seem to be in a muddle about 'treatment'. Today we also have a situation where people's everyday problems are being medicalised.

Treatment is often with anti-depressants or other mood-altering drugs. Take sadness as an example. Sadness is part of being human – just as happiness is – it is not an illness. There could be a perfectly rational explanation for your sadness – for instance grief at the loss of a loved one or fear about the ramifications of losing one's income after redundancy. Taking a course of anti-depressants is not necessarily the only answer.

This is not to deny the very real condition of clinical depression but just to point out that there are many occasions when medications are being used as a first port of call or as a long-term habitual fix. Becoming unemployed, for instance, can lead to a person being anxious and downhearted. Arguably the solution for most people is a suitable job not an anti-depressant. Likewise, with the menopause or a messy divorce – the solution is often to be found in good support systems – friends, mentors, trusty legal, financial and mediation advisers.

Stress – do you need it?

So to address today's number one monster – 'stress'. Without a certain level of stress, as an arousal mechanism, life would be tedious and somewhat pointless – as the saying goes 'variety is the spice of life'. It transpires that an optimum level of stress arousal is a pre-requisite for personal and professional growth. For example, that talk you volunteered to give at your local community centre, or your annual work assessment presentation to your boss, may have made you feel extremely stressed, but it also allowed you to accomplish something worthwhile.

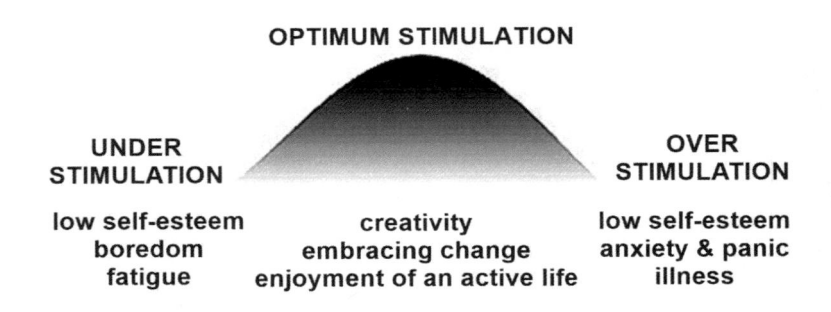

UNDER STIMULATION	OPTIMUM STIMULATION	OVER STIMULATION
low self-esteem	creativity	low self-esteem
boredom	embracing change	anxiety & panic
fatigue	enjoyment of an active life	illness

By way of contrast, at the top end of the scale, too much stress creates physiological tension and your body goes haywire, causing a predisposition to 'ill-being'. Is the solution a pill from your doctor or a change of circumstances, a different attitude, priority scheduling, physical activity, an emotional overhaul, a relaxing holiday, an escapist book or movie? Or all of these?

The happy medium

Whatever your illness or wellness issues, only you know the best way to find the happy medium that balances the many factors impacting your precious health. By making changes at home to present a supportive Habitat Affect, you can establish healthier physical and emotional habits – helpful things you can do for yourself, and for your friends, your family and the wider world.

"Be really whole and all things will come to you." Lao-Tzu.

8. MIND MATTERS – LUCK – 100% NOW

"Attitude is a little thing that makes a big difference." Winston Churchill. If someone asked you to describe your 'frame of mind' what would you say? Optimistic or pessimistic? Curious or closed off? Thoughtful? Variable, depending on the situation?

There are certain mind-sets that make it easier for us to function well, even during difficult times, while others tend to bring us down and reinforce helplessness. To quote Dennis Brown: *"The only difference between a good day and a bad day is your attitude."*

One way of getting to know the nature of your mind better is to practice meditation. In the 8th Enrichment Experience [Part 2] Action Area there are specific instructions about an insightful, and increasingly popular, form of meditation called 'Mindfulness'. There is also an overview of Mindfulness in Appendix D. For now we take a look at some general aspects of the human mind and marvel at its ability to provide daily experiences through the choices we make – choices which can be supported by Habitat Affect cues – Focus Features – around our homes.

Open-minded and curious

'Keep an open mind' is a popular piece of advice. Being curious – open to the novel and the unexplored – keeps life fresh and invigorating. If your habit is rigidly entrenched in a particular way of looking at the world, you may miss out on all sorts of experiences.

Ask yourself if you have fixed views and opinions on lots of things or are you flexible and free in your mode of thought? Can you see the other person's point of view, even if you don't agree with it? Do you compromise when necessary for a mutually beneficial result? Are you a good listener? Can you acknowledge when you don't know something without embarrassment? According to mystic Thomas Merton: what really matters is openness, courage and giving attention where it is due.

Open-minded people are not afraid to think outside the box, to try new things, change their minds, compromise, re-schedule when necessary, laugh at their mistakes and be spontaneous. There is even a physical side to being open-minded – it is reflected in a relaxed body stance, a head held up high and friendly eye contact. Remember this when you look in the mirror – and smile!

Learning to be more open

In the relatively new field of Positive Psychology, the term 'learned helplessness' describes a close-minded state where people become unable to cope in a receptive, productive and open-minded way. For a variety of reasons, they become victims of their own misfortune and let life 'happen' to them. Physically they may fold their arms, bow their heads, avoid eye contact – they are unhappy.

Fortunately, people can change their outlook by resilience training in 'learned optimism' which naturally involves being curious and open-minded. The 3rd Enrichment Experience mentions ways to create a personal Habitat Affect that inspires learning and curiosity. In the meantime, you are encouraged to identify any habits – either in your thinking, in your speech or in your actions – that may be preventing you from being open-minded and ready to seize the moment. As Einstein said: *"the important thing is not to stop questioning"*.

Attitude health check

"Our progress in life is equal to our capacity to let go of our problems and move ahead with the momentum of a positive attitude." Karen Casey & Martha Vanceburg. Are you a person whose glass is half full or half empty? What is your current attitude towards the most important people and situations in your life? Having a bright 'can-do' attitude bodes well for health and happiness but it is not always that easy in today's highly competitive busy stressful world.

Attitude is rooted in the deeply cherished beliefs we hold about ourselves – our hopes and dreams, our capabilities and our passions. 'That's all very well' you may say, but what about feelings of fear, doubt, anxiety and uncertainty? At an extreme, after experiencing personal tragedy, most people's ability to cope well is quite appropriately dampened for a considerable while. Perversely, even when there are no disturbing issues, having an entrenched attitude may subconsciously bring a victim mentality into play, possibly self-sabotage or some other familiar behaviour, despite the fact that such negativity can result in a poor outcome.

Moving to a 'can-do' attitude

Psychologists have a Theory of Cognitive Dissonance which suggests that if you behave in a certain way, your thoughts and beliefs will eventually change to conform to your behaviour. This has been shown to work in the fraught area of overcoming prejudices. For instance, if someone who identifies as 'a glass half empty person' deliberately decides to behave – that is, actually 'to do' something actively – in a positive 'can-do' manner, then after a while their underlying attitude will shift accordingly to justify their actions.

You can try this for yourself by the simple act of smiling when you are feeling down. Say the phrase 'smile for health' out loud before each smile. See what happens.

In the book 'Life of Pi' by Yann Martel, Pi says: *"The spot was in fact no different from when I had passed it not long before, but my way of seeing it had changed."* Think about this sentence metaphorically and try to apply it to an incident in your own life where a change of attitude might deliver a different perspective on the episode in question.

Harness your 'luck energy attitude'

There is a saying *'you make your own luck'*. A dictionary definition of luck is 'success or failure apparently brought by chance'. However, we all know that some people seem to be 'born lucky' and some are downright unlucky – could it be that there is more to this than mere chance?

It may well be that on occasion our experience of 'luck' is linked to the subtle energy – either positive, negative or neutral – that we give out. This subtle energy is intrinsic to our feelings, our attitude, our tone of voice, our facial expression, our body language – any or all of which seem to attract similar energy.

Forget for a moment the traditional western meaning of luck as being something which happens completely by chance. Consider instead that when we put out positive energy to the universe, to our friends and family, even to people we are not overly enamoured with, then we, in turn, attract positive things to ourselves.

Even when something apparently negative happens, we can choose to use it to our advantage. There may be a lesson that we need to learn for our future well-being or we may entertain the thought that 'if this had not happened, then something worse was around the corner', so we have been saved from it. How about giving this way of thinking – this 'luck energy attitude' – a whirl for the next week or so? With any luck, you will be able to notice how lucky you are!

Sensational animals

Our chances of what appears to be 'good luck' can also increase if we tap into the world of animal senses. Animals and birds can detect an impending tsunami and leave for higher ground, way ahead of the approaching deluge. If you were party to this information, you could follow their lead which some might call 'a lucky escape'.

Dogs are well known for their ability to sense the minutest changes in energy – witness the response of a family pet when there is anger around – tail instantly between hind legs. Dogs can be trained to assist people with epilepsy because they can sense an imminent seizure. Likewise, they can detect the presence of cancer in a person before the medical team has made a firm diagnosis. Someone with such a dog would indeed be 'lucky' to get early treatment.

Eliminating pessimism

Helen Keller, a deaf blind author and political activist, said: *"No pessimist ever discovered the secret of the stars or sailed to an uncharted land."* So if you believe that you are going to fail at something, your repressed 'can't-do' approach expresses 'negativity' and, in this poor energy environment, an unfavourable outcome is far more likely.

'It's just my bad luck' you may say – 'yes' you are probably going to fail, just like you thought you would. However, if you believe that you are going to succeed, even if the outcome is not quite as you expected, your 'can-do' bright energy attracts 'good luck' and you are far more likely to enjoy a favourable result.

We encourage you to think of ways in which you can make your home environment a haven for 'good luck' energy to circulate and lift your spirits.

Memory and reality

As you come to understand your own mind and emotions better, you will be more comfortable with the idea that 'reality' is not quite what it seems – more detail on 'reality' in the 8th Enrichment Experience. An appreciation of the complex nature of 'reality' is most helpful when it comes to communicating with other people – robust interpersonal relationships are vital for our happiness and well-being.

Everything you think and do is relative to your particular circumstances and mindset, including your memory, which can be an extraordinarily fickle friend! This means that what you think of as your reality is not necessarily someone else's reality. Nonetheless you can do your very best to accept responsibility for 'telling it like it is' [diplomatically], whenever possible. If you do this, your life will be much more straightforward and ultimately enjoyable.

Most of us, from time to time, allow a devious persona to surface, embellishing the truth about what really happened – we call this 'glamorising' our memory. These are the stories we tell ourselves, and others, to justify our thoughts and actions – the stories we may even come to believe are a true version of reality if frequently repeated enough.

Glamorising memory

Most often our glamorising is just a slight deviation from what we are actually thinking and doing, making our position more acceptable. Glamorising may also appear to gain us someone's approval that we desperately crave, or help to re-invent our life stories for a completely fresh start. Whatever our purpose, the glamorised version of events can be a useful catalyst to help us feel better about the past.

Remember the good old days? Recall that photo of you where you looked gorgeous but were actually seething inside? Sometimes even vivid dreams appear so real that they become part of your memory, as if they actually happened.

Glamorised memories can be very convincing. By acknowledging that there is a tendency to glamorise life experiences [as many of us do], you can begin to recognise 'the way things really are' – a major tenet of Buddhist philosophy – then real benefits follow.

Can you recall a recent incident when you slightly embellished the facts? If so, take an objective look [from the outside as if you are someone else] and try to understand what was really going on. You may find this experience an opportunity to learn about how the stories we tell ourselves influence the outcomes we experience. *"… it's no secret that the past proves a most unstable mirror, typically too severe and flattering all at once, and never as truth-reflecting as people would like to believe."* Chang-Rae Lee

The 'now' experience

There is a lot of talk these days about 'living in the moment', the now, the present. This may give the impression that the past and the future are of no concern, which can be confusing.

Most of us know what it is like to have 'a chattering mind' filled with thoughts about the past and expectations about the future, while the present moment is gone in a flash. In a very real sense, your mind tends to operate as the link between your memories and your projections about what might happen in future. What then of the present moment?

Well the present moment is actually about 'experience'. And experience embodies your motivations and intentions which create your future experiences. While you may draw on memories and hopes to colour your experience, the actual act of experiencing can only ever be in the present moment.

Perhaps you would like to take 'this moment' to think about your concept of what it means to be aware of the present – awake to the here and now. You will probably discover that it is far easier to think back over the past or dream about the future, than it is to focus on the present moment.

Looked at from a different perspective, if you continually find yourself focusing on past memories or future hopes at the expense of truly experiencing whatever is happening in the present, then you are likely to be living a 'half-life'. In such a half-life situation, you deny yourself the opportunity to enjoy fully your actual life as it plays out right here – right now.

100% present for shining moments

Thich Nhat Hanh, an astute Vietnamese Buddhist monk, has some helpful advice. He suggests concentrating fully and giving 100% effort to whatever it is that you choose to be thinking or doing in any given moment – without distraction.

Try it for yourself – even if you are doing something that might normally seem to be a chore like cleaning the house, preparing food or visiting an elderly relative who is unable to hold an intelligent conversation. You will be amazed at how much better you feel when giving your full attention to the job in hand. Your mind relaxes as it lets go of the past and future, and expands into the present moment.

You can always employ a mindfulness technique to help you stay focused. For example, think about the miracle of the food you are preparing – work out its origins, right back to the planting of a seed, nourished by water and sunlight. If you are conversing with an elderly infirm person, really listen to what they are saying and when it is your turn to respond, be mindful of the words and phrases you use to cheer them.

We recommend that you try to fill your days with as many 'shining moment' experiences as you can, one moment at a time. *"As you walk and eat and travel, be where you are. Otherwise you will miss most of your life."* Buddha.

9. ACTIONS SPEAK LOUDER THAN WORDS

"Until one is committed, there is hesitancy, the chance to draw back . . . Concerning all acts of initiative and creation, there is one elementary truth that, ignorance of which, kills countless ideas and splendid plans: that the moment one definitely commits oneself, then providence moves too. All sorts of things occur to help one that would never otherwise have occurred. A whole stream of events issues from the decision, raising in one's favour all manner of unforeseen incidents and meetings and material assistance, which nobody could have dreamed would have come their way. Whatever you can do, or dream you can do, begin it. Boldness has genius, power, and magic in it. Begin it now." This saying is often attributed to Goethe but variations are evident from several previous and following authors.

By being committed to act, you are poised to create your very own Habitat Affect by introducing personal Focus Features – 'action reminders' which can influence your physical, mental and emotional well-being. According to Jean-Paul Sartre: *"Commitment is an act, not a word."* Each of the 9 Enrichment Experiences in Part 2 includes guidance on appropriate acts – you choose to commit to the ones that are in resonance with your individual circumstances.

As your actions produce 'experiences', you are gifted with outcomes which provide opportunities to learn and grow in knowledge and wisdom. Even if a particular outcome is not quite what you initially had in mind – it can be seen as a lesson in life that will influence your upcoming choices, allowing you to be more 'successful' in the future.

What does success look like for you?

Putting things in perspective, you may like to ponder, and possibly add to, the following descriptions of success.

Success is loving others; allowing myself to be loved; using my natural kindness and compassion well; helping to bring out the best in people; earning the respect of other people by example.

Success is being true to myself and my chosen values; having the courage to rise above fear of failure; learning a better way from my mistakes; seizing opportunities for healthy new experiences; giving appropriately and unconditionally of my time and of my surplus funds; knowing when enough is enough.

Success is finding time to play, to have fun, to smile and laugh; spending time with children and the elderly; appreciating beauty and the simple things of life. Finally, when it is time for me to leave this world, knowing that someone somewhere has benefited from something I have contributed – however small or seemingly insignificant.

Harnessing the ability to focus and to receive

In order to create fresh insights, new skills and rewarding experiences, you will need both the ability to focus your attention as necessary, and room in your mind to allow these new things to come into your life.

Here are some useful questions. Are you currently full to bursting or an empty vessel? Are you so busy that your chattering mind gets clogged up? Do you allow information overload to swamp your thinking – constant smartphone interaction, emails, facebook, twitter, blogs, youtube, instagram, newspapers, magazines? Do you feel anxious if you haven't checked out the latest this or that? Would you like to 'fast your frenzy' at least some of the time and be ready to receive rather different life experiences?

There's an ancient Taoist saying 'the empty vessel is ready to receive' which is illustrated by a story about a wise teacher Master How-So and an apparently knowledgeable man Mr. Too, who was 'too full up' to take advantage of the opportunities in his life for happiness. You can read this seemingly quaint story in Appendix E; it is thought-provoking on several levels.

Determined resolve

Of course, being committed to action – making wise choices on a day-to-day basis – does require sustained effort. Yet it is through your effort, and sometimes struggle, that the reward of a worthwhile life is to be found. St Francis of Assisi is reputed to have said *"The reward of patience is patience."* To parody this, we say that *'the reward of engaging in the 9 Enrichments is the 9 Enrichments'*.

So give yourself the green light to make your life-changing intentions come to fruition. Action without deliberate resolve is a waste of time; we can only make real long-term life changes when we are personally ready to do so – not just because we thought it was 'the right thing', 'about time' or because we 'read it in a book'.

Sometimes people have to hit 'rock bottom' before they realise that things cannot continue as they have without serious consequences. Rock bottom, gazing into the abyss of hopelessness, is an extremely uncomfortable, sometimes life-threatening, place and best avoided at all costs. If you are feeling overwhelmingly downcast 'now' is the time to take action. There is always potential for a brighter future.

Of course you may already have a fulfilling life and simply want to make even better use of your time and energy.

Whatever your circumstances, determined resolve to make healthy choices – slowly yet surely – is the way forward.

If you have read this far, and want to continue your personal quest today – 'the first day of the rest of your life' – the next step is to develop your personal Habitat Affect via the 9 Enrichments Experience. *"The secret of success is to be ready when your opportunity comes."* Disraeli.

PART 2

EXPERIENCING THE HABITAT AFFECT

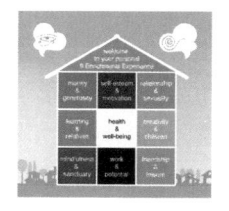

THE 1st ENRICHMENT EXPERIENCE

Work; career; vocation; volunteering; using your skills; releasing hidden potential; consolidation of ideas; planning; hibernation; the seed waiting in the ground. *"Happiness does not come from doing easy work but from the afterglow of satisfaction with the achievement of a difficult task that demanded our best."* Theodore Isaac Rubin.

We spend a significant part of our lives either working, thinking about work or, if we're out of a job, trying to find employment that marries with our circumstances and our passions. From the depression of unemployment or the daily grind of monotonous tasks to the sheer joy of loving every working moment, our job, career or occupation – call it what you will – does seem to matter a great deal to most of us. Indeed it may be used to define who we profess to be when in conversation with others.

Some people love their work, others see it as a source of tension and stress. Finding a balance between work and family life can be difficult. Aspiring business executives may feel they need 'to be seen to be working long hours'. Then there's the army of people who are fooled into thinking that being 'busily busy' is smart. For stay-at-home Mums or Dads, there can be the feeling that the house-keeping role needs to be justified.

Recently retired workers can get stuck as they search for something meaningful to keep them occupied and feeling useful. For those people who have been made redundant, work is suddenly a massive issue. Finding yourself unexpectedly out of work can be extremely scary, yet it can also be a time for some serious re-evaluation and an opportunity for a different work experience.

What's your work story, your work ethic, your vocational passion, your hidden potential, your volunteering aspiration? This is what you are here to explore and to celebrate in the 1st Enrichment Experience. You might like to start by identifying your work type, the amount of time you spend at work and whether or not this suits your well-being.

Your current work situation

Broadly speaking, 'work type' can be categorised as follows. Identify the group or groups appropriate to you:

paid 'career' employment based outside the home
paid 'career' employment working from home
paid job based outside the home – full time
paid job based outside the home – part time
paid job working from home – full time
paid job working from home – part-time
temporary paid job based outside the home – full time
temporary paid job based outside the home – part time
temporary paid job working from home – full time
temporary paid job working from home – part time
voluntary unpaid work based outside the home
voluntary unpaid work based at home
'unpaid' work in the home – housework
'unpaid' work in the home – childrearing
overtime work to supplement income
unemployed looking for work
unemployed on short-term training scheme
unemployed on disability benefits
studying full time
studying part time
other .... please specify.

Does your current work type suit you and sustain your ambitions? If not, how would you like to progress? What is your ideal work type – in 1 year – in 3 years – in 5 years?

Time spent on the job

If 'time at work' is an issue for you, then how about making a few constructive changes to address this? To set the context for change, perhaps start by making an assessment of the amount of time that you currently devote to work on a weekly basis. "On average I spend approximately XX hours a week on work plus YY hours on work-related thoughts." You may also want to elaborate on time spent doing housework, particularly if you find this hard to fit into your schedule, or if there are issues around the division of labour in a shared home environment.

What does your personal work/life balance look like? Is it in keeping with your age and stage? Are you happy with the amount of time your work takes? It's a longstanding joke but well worth repeating: when did you ever hear anyone on their deathbed gasp "oh how I wish I'd spent more time at the office"?

All work involves 'your lifetime', so it is healthy if you can regard work as an enjoyable way to spend part of that time. Your work can keep you involved and active – mentally and physically. It can give you a sense of accomplishment and purpose. It can promote feelings of self-worth that underpin your confidence and ability to engage with others. Depending on your type of employment, your position and relationship with colleagues, work can sometimes provide opportunities for pleasurable social activities as well.

If you are experiencing difficulties at work or find that your work/life balance is out of kilter, then maybe it is time to make a few changes, but what do those changes look like?

Reality check for work change

You might decide to re-think your attitude, behaviour and time vis-à-vis your current work pattern or make a radical change and enter a new field of occupation. Always remember that 'the you at work' is affected by all the other facets of your life, so please keep an open-minded approach to your thinking.

Being open-minded is particularly important if your livelihood has been affected by the worldwide economic downturn. We are not pretending that it is going to be easy if you have been made redundant and are struggling financially and emotionally. However, we are suggesting that if you face the challenge of this unexpected situation with a constructive attitude, you are more likely to find another job or even a new career path.

One other thing to mention briefly: it may become apparent that 'the problem' is not your problem but, for instance, that of your boss or the organisational culture in which you find yourself.

Once you understand that even if you were to make changes yourself, the problem would not go away, you may need to take a different approach. Perhaps you could ask to be transferred to another department? Or maybe you could investigate the possibility of leaving your present employment and starting afresh?

Think through all options carefully and avoid jeopardising your present position by being loose tongued. Making changes at work requires diplomacy and personal integrity. If you have responsibility for financially supporting other people, then any changes must be particularly well planned.

Am I employing my skills to the full?

Whatever your particular scenario, it always feels good to know that your talents and skills are being used to the full, rather than being wasted. Yet, so often, untapped potential can remain hidden and never realised. If you find yourself in the 'untapped potential zone', remember that there is always scope for something extra or different, maybe expanding your job, volunteering or travelling or all three.

The 1st Enrichment is all about optimising your potential, bringing those latent talents out into the open and truly enjoying what you do, in keeping with your physical, mental and spiritual well-being.

As you enter the following ACTION AREA, be encouraged by this upbeat saying *"We are all potentially heroes and geniuses if only we would have the courage, and do the hard work, necessary to becoming so."* Unamuno.

The 1st Enrichment Experience Action Area

The following ACTIONS A-D are a pick 'n' mix of work-related ideas for you to try. They can help you discover your working patterns and determine what choices-for-change, if any, would enrich your work experience and your voluntary activities. ACTION B specifically relates to things you can do to optimise the Habitat Affect in your home. Select the actions that feel right for your circumstances, ignore the rest.

ACTION A: Questions & answers – your motivating letter

Write yourself a personal letter [Dear Me . . . and the date] in which you answer one or more of the following questions:

Thinking about your work, are you generally content with your current situation or is there anything obvious that you'd like to change immediately. If so, how?

Thinking about your work and your future prospects what would you like to happen over the next 3-5 years? What do you need to do to make this happen?

Are you happy with your work/life balance – if not, how would you like to change it?

As you write your letter, you may find that some of your answers point to the need for fairly significant change. Yet, even if several aspects of your working life need to be reviewed, be confident that you will be able to deal with them over time.

Perhaps your answers indicate some kind of change in your attitude, your working habits, the need to seek promotion, desire for a new job or an entirely different career path? If any of these scenarios resonates with you, are there any obvious pointers as to where you could realistically start to initiate choices-for-change? Be constructive so that your letter avoids negativity and is one of positive intention. You can add to it anytime.

Headline your final paragraph with the words "Glad to be alive." Now choose three things, related in some way to the 1st Enrichment, that 'make your heart sing'. They might be people, situations or objects in your working life for which you are grateful, unexpected things that have happened out of the blue or golden opportunities opening up. An easy way to do this is to finish the sentence: "I'm glad that I …….."

Put your completed letter into an envelope [preferably blue or white] and place it in the north of your home or workplace. The significance of this will become apparent in ACTION B.

ACTION B: Create an inspiring environment

"The space in which I work is a reflection of myself – do I respect that space?" Imagine that your workplace is as you would expect to find in a highly successful global company – could you develop it accordingly?

Traditionally rooms with a northerly aspect are considered very auspicious for the work ethic – here sunlight is experienced indirectly through reflection. The north is considered to represent stable energy – cool reflection and the consolidation of ideas – a place to engage calmly and strategically with your work.

However, each of the compass directions has a role to play in 'the you at work' because everything is interconnected. Therefore, if your office is in the south it will help to fire you up for action, while an eastern-sited workplace is good for learning and a western one for completing projects. Whatever your workstation compass position – pay special attention to its north-facing aspect as described in 'Focus Features – placing on purpose – physical reminders' below.

The same goes if you are currently unemployed and looking for work. Choose an area of your home in which to honour your work ethic and decorate it with colours and items that are symbolic of the opportunities you wish to secure, following the advice for workplaces that follows.

Purge your workplace for productivity

It is easier to think clearly, stay focused and achieve tasks when your surroundings are organised and non-distractive – messy without, so within. As well as ugly clutter, even the display of excess objects and possessions in your workplace can be a hindrance. It is worth asking if the things you see around you are nurturing and encouraging of clear thinking and dedicated activity?

You can choose to clear away anything that is stale or cluttering up your workplace. The best way to purge is to take out every moveable object [including books, files, pictures, worktop mess etc] and then gradually re-introduce each one, asking the questions: is this really necessary and, if so, where should it be displayed or stored attractively? This will force you to organise your work equipment, papers and other items in an aesthetically pleasing way. There really is no need to have ugly piles of 'stuff' around.

Organising – your surroundings and computer filing system

Perhaps you already have a storage system that helps you achieve a smooth-running, physically appealing workplace? However, if that is not the case, then it is worth taking a little time to decide on the kind of system that would suit your working type and job requirements for both filing and discarding information when it arrives. In other words, get your information handling systems and storage organised so it is easy to sustain a great working environment – that goes for e-storage on your computer as well.

If you identify the need for more storage, develop an easy-to-use system without delay. We are great fans of having good shelving and plenty of box files in which to store hard copy items. But you must find the right solution for you – all we can do is exhort you to go right ahead and install it.

Focus Features – placing on purpose – physical reminders

If you like, you can introduce some specific placements, rearrangements, décor changes – your Focus Features – that have positive, possibly symbolic, meaning for you. Your Focus Features will act as very real physical reminders of your chosen path for future success and enjoyment of your working life. Here are some ideas and suggestions, they are not meant to be prescriptive, just do what feels good for you:

- When sitting in your working position, it is best to have a solid wall behind you and a good view of the entrance. Sitting with your back to the door is not the most productive arrangement. A basic biological survival mechanism means your mind is subconsciously on red alert in case someone sneaks up behind you which may detract from your ability to concentrate fully.

- Imagine your office chair is a throne and empower yourself! Place a picture of a mountain or other robust supportive image on the wall behind you. Place a motivating image that represents your goals on the wall you see from your desk. For example, if your business is global, or aspires to be, then a world map may work well for you. If you are a garden designer, then a picture of a beautiful garden or a plant would be in keeping. An image of whatever symbolises success in your working life will encourage your endeavours.

- Make sure that your posture at work is mechanically good for your spine and shoulders, particularly if you are working on a computer all day or lifting heavy weights – goods or people. If you are mainly a sedentary worker, remember to take frequent standing/walking breaks – post a 'Focus Feature reminder' in your work station. Also ensure your working area is well illuminated. Do you have access to natural daylight? Fresh air? If not, please make sure these two aspects are factored into your work breaks. If there is a company gym, use it!

- If you have a choice, then the north of a building is considered to be a good place for an office location with its cool reflected light and connection with the flow of the water element. Even if your office is located elsewhere, you can 'honour the north' with one or two Focus Features. You can place a glass bowl here – glass is symbolic of water, as are the colours blue and black. The bowl can either be a reminder of the empty vessel ready to receive [see Appendix E], or you may like to place your work-related letter [ACTION A above] in the bowl or you can write a short wish list of work-related aims and place it here.

- Place any objects in the north that symbolise work success and enjoyment. A vase of fresh blue flowers will enhance the energy for clear thinking. The north is also a good place to display work-related certificates or trophies. For fun, an ornamental tortoise placed in the north can help you to remember the story of the hare and the tortoise and who eventually won the race!

- Colours should be thought through carefully if you have a choice in the matter. Each colour has a different effect, so your colour scheme should depend on the nature of your work, your individual work style and your personality [please see Appendix D for colour attributes]. For instance, blue aids logical thought and clarity of information, yellow is good for 'mood' communications, pale green can provide an ideal learning environment, purple is creative, orange is said to be sociable. Silver and gold are solid and robust with promises of travel and helpful friends. White reflects all possibilities. If you need to boost self-confidence and keep 'fired up' then introduce some red, but in moderation – an excess can act as a stress-arousal mechanism. You can introduce red in the form of a red flowering plant or vase of flowers, a red baize desktop or notice board, a red paperweight or mouse mat. How about a red tablet/laptop?

- Your working life is associated with the water element which is useful if something or someone at work triggers your anger. Before 'reacting' [particularly before pressing send on an angry text, email or twitter feed etc], come to the cool reflective north. Here you can spend a few moments in which to breathe deeply and think through a wise course of responsive action or non-action – the calming effect of this northerly direction is immediate.

- Today our computerised workplaces are electrically charged environments that might be regarded as unhealthy. The presence of broad-leaved plants has been shown by NASA to help counter electro-magnetic pollution. We recommend that you keep a plant on or near your desk. Make sure any plants you have at work are thriving and tend them well for best performance. If you work in an artificially illuminated office, you may need to change your plant quite often.

ACTION C: The 3 column tracker exercise

Stuck in a rut? Feeling unfulfilled? Not sure which direction to take in your working/charitable life? Then try 'The 3 column tracker' exercise which has been designed to help you find direction and fulfilment.

Take a sheet of lined paper landscape and rule 2 vertical lines so that you end up with three equal columns.

[1] Head the first column 'Things I'm good at'. Underneath write down absolutely everything you are good at. Start with vocation-related talents and then list anything that you personally do well, be it cleaning or woodwork, arranging flowers, singing, cooking, organising a sports team etc.

[2] Head the second column 'Things I'm qualified to do'. By qualified, we mean both academic qualifications and things that you have been doing for so long that you are considered to be expertly knowledgeable.

[3] Head the third column 'Things I absolutely love doing'. The title of this column speaks for itself. As with the first column, do not restrict yourself merely to vocational exploits.

Interpretation

We expect you have already noticed that some things appear in more than one column. If something appears in all three columns, then you have a clear marker for the direction in which you will find fulfilment. However, if you only have a two column link, we suggest you consider only those items which occur in the third column and one other. This is because it is unlikely you will experience happiness and a sense of achievement long-term from doing things that you don't feel passionate about.

Life is not a dress rehearsal, so you might as well try to optimise your opportunities for doing things that you really enjoy, even as part of your working regime. If this exercise indicates the possibility of a radical job change, then you may have to do some additional training.

If you are responsible for financially supporting dependents, then ensure the timing of any training doesn't jeopardise your ability to meet their needs. Obviously the welfare of young children is paramount, but that doesn't mean you can't organise some evening classes or an online college course, of which there are now thousands to choose from.

Whatever you decide, be it charity work, a completely new career or just asking your boss in a constructive way for promotion, we wish you a rewarding result.

ACTION D: Make a difference – change something

This is your chance to make a stated commitment to change something for the better. You could just commit to a general change in attitude and belief about work. Better still, you could detail a specific goal and the practical actions necessary to achieve it in an organised and enjoyable way.

If you set yourself a working goal, it needs to be stated as a positive intention – for example "to spend less time at work" is a hazy phrase. In this case your target could read something like "to spend a sensible amount of time at work vis-à-vis my other life activities" – and specify a weekly average target. If you are actively seeking work, the more specific you can be about your goals, the better.

As with the option of writing a letter to yourself in Action A, you can write down your motivating goal and the steps you need to take to get there. Place your written goal in the north of your home or workplace.

Work well and be well for work

Whatever you choose to change relating to your work, make sure it is in tune with the essence of the 1st Enrichment – that is to enhance the enjoyment of your working life by using your skills and talents to the full.

THE 2nd ENRICHMENT EXPERIENCE

Personal relationships; love; romance; sexual intimacy; expressing desire; compromise; companionship; the joy of sharing; being contently single; looking for a soulmate. *"Keep love in your heart. A life without it is like a sunless garden when the flowers are dead. The consciousness of loving and being loved brings a warmth and richness to life that nothing else can bring."* Oscar Wilde.

The 2nd Enrichment Experience is all about personal relationships – yours with your partner or the desire to meet a like-minded partner or being comfortable on your own for a while or deciding that being happily single is your permanent favoured option. Please note that you will have a chance to consider your relationships with parents, children, family members and friends while exploring other enrichments.

For those of you who currently embrace a shared love life, this is a chance to re-fresh aspects of your relationship or to make essential changes. Others of you may be seeking to enter a new partnership or support yourself in the pleasure of being contently single which brings its own set of benefits.

Two people – one relationship

Because personal relationships necessarily involve two people, there will always be a need for sharing, for compromise and for compassion. And always remember – there is no such thing as 'the perfect relationship'. So please be prepared to accommodate the other person's feelings and failings, as well as their fabulousness!

One thing we can definitely say: there is no point in being in a relationship unless you both make an effort to ensure the experience is mutually beneficial. This includes making up well after a row and being able to laugh together. It is also worth considering that 'the you in relationship' is affected by all the other facets of your life, so each of the 9 Enrichments has a role in strengthening your loving persona.

Sensitive communication

Siegfried Sassoon wrote *"Words are fools, who follow blindly once they get a lead. But thoughts are kingfishers that haunt the pools of quiet, seldom seen."* The words we use in relationships, and the things that we sometimes refrain from saying, are a key part of living harmoniously with a partner.

Our choice of words has massive consequences for the health of a personal relationship or during the phase when we are trying to connect with a new partner. Words often provide the medium through which we meet each other's emotional needs and demonstrate our appreciation. Words are very powerful – once spoken it is impossible to 'unsay' the words, so we need to make sure they are the ones we really mean to use.

'Skill-full' speech has long been recognised in Buddhist teachings as a primer for healthy dialogue and communication that avoids knowingly causing distress. Never is this more so than in our personal relationships, where an angry word or a selfish revelation can cause such long-term damage. On the other hand, an encouraging word from a loved one is like sunshine on a grey day.

We all know how easy it is to lose verbal control in the heat of the moment, especially with our nearest and dearest. This is why we need to find 'a speech brake' [a deep breath maybe?], that allows us to stop the flow and re-phrase in mutually helpful language. Just thinking about the words, phrases and tone of voice that we use to communicate, can help us to see where subtle changes might make a massive difference to the nature of our relationship.

The phrase 'abracadabra' comes from the ancient Aramaic 'abraq ad habra' which literally means 'I will create as I speak'. If you are trying to say something sensitive to your partner, it may help to imagine you are waving a magic wand over yourself and use 'abracadabra' to find the right words – the words that will create the outcome you both need for harmony.

Sexual compatibility

So many factors affect the success or otherwise of a personal relationship, but it is fair to say that compatibility on sexual matters is important for most couples. Frequency of love-making, trust in faithfulness and acceptable types of sexual coupling, are all factors. Whether you make love once a day, once a week or once a month – it is best you both agree, more or less, on frequency, with the option of spontaneity. Likewise, regarding sexual practices, you both need to feel they are appropriate for your relationship.

However sexual compatibility is something of a chicken and egg situation. When there is an apparent problem between the two of you, is it the other niggles in the relationship that are causing difficulty with the sexual relationship? Or is it the lack of sexual harmony that appears to underlie tension and problems in other departments?

It is perhaps appropriate to mention that you won't find any explicit sexual advice in this book – the mechanics of sex and articles about what a good time everyone else seems to be having are always available from the thousands of publications, films and websites currently around. The Habitat Affect 2nd Enrichment Experience is designed specifically to help you make happy healthy choices that co-join the experience of sex and love.

NB. Anyone reading this who has been in an abusive sexual relationship or in a relationship with a member of his or her own family or is anxious or depressed should seek professional help.

Love and romance

That loaded word 'love' – it means different things to different people so it is really helpful to be clear about what you mean when you use the word 'love' with regard to an intimate personal relationship – think about this for a moment. Understanding the nature of your love and how to keep love alive is a beautiful thing of which to be mindful. We are quoting Sonnet 116 by Shakespeare as being a wonderful interpretation of the nature of true love:

> Let me not to the marriage of true minds
>
> Admit impediments. Love is not love
>
> Which alters when it alteration finds,
>
> Or bends with the remover to remove:
>
> Oh, no! It is an ever-fixed mark,
>
> That looks on tempests and is never shaken;
>
> It is the star to every wandering bark,
>
> Whose worth's unknown, although his height be taken.
>
> Love's not time's fool, though rosy lips and cheeks
>
> Within his bending sickle's compass come;
>
> Love alters not with his brief hours and weeks,
>
> But bears it out even to the edge of doom.
>
> If this be error, and upon me proved,
>
> I never writ, nor no man ever loved.

We uphold that 'true love' is constant and long-term, while 'falling in love' is a genetic-biochemical mechanism – sometimes labelled as 'lust' – to ensure that we, as a species, reproduce. As we all know, this falling in love phase passes but hopefully matures into special mutually adoring companionship love with a satisfying sexual element.

So how do you keep love alive in a long-term relationship? In Appendix F – Keeping love alive – we've come up with a list of '10 golden guidelines' based on romance psychology, personal experience and that of our friends. And if you are single, a couple of our suggestions may be helpful when you are thinking of dating or trying to establish a partnership.

The 2nd Enrichment Experience Action Area

The following ACTIONS A-D are a pick 'n' mix of relationship-related ideas to help you appreciate your personal relationship patterns and see what choices-for-change, if any, you might consider to enrich your love life. ACTION B specifically relates to things you can do to optimise the Habitat Affect in your home. Select the actions that feel right for your circumstances, ignore the others.

ACTION A: Questions & answers – your motivating letter

Write a personal letter [Dear Me or Dear Us, plus the date], in which you answer one or more of the following questions:

If you are in a life-long partnership, are you generally content with the current situation and your future prospects?

Is there anything obvious that you would like to change immediately or over the longer-term?

If you are single, for whatever reason, are you happily single or would you like to share your life with someone and, if so, what sort of relationship would you like?

As you write your letter, you may find that some of your answers indicate the potential for a few beneficial changes. If so, ask yourself and your partner, as appropriate, to discuss these opportunities and write about them. Always try to be constructive so that your letter avoids negativity and is one of positive intention. You can add to it anytime.

Headline your final paragraph: "Glad to be alive." Now choose three things, related to the 2nd Enrichment, that 'make your heart sing'. If you are in a relationship, they might be quirky things about your partner that make you laugh, satisfying things that you do together such as travel or making a beautiful garden, or those romantic gestures for which you are grateful. An easy way to do this is to finish the sentence: "I'm glad that ……..". Alternatively, if you are looking for a relationship, focus on the attributes you can bring to a partnership and mention the opportunities you have for meeting new people: "I'm glad that I can ……..". In both cases, end your letter with this beautiful quote from Aristotle: "*To love is to rejoice.*"

Now put your completed letter in an envelope [preferably the colour of your favourite gem stone], and place it in the south west of your home. The significance of this will become apparent in ACTION B.

ACTION B: Create an inspiring environment

The places we associate with romance and personal relationships are many and varied. However to generalise, we are going to mention: the gorgeous bedroom, the large seductive sofa, the table where you might share a sexy eating experience, the exercise gym where you sweat together, the back row of the movies where you hold hands, the south west of your home. You may not have been expecting a compass direction, yet we ask you to be open-minded to the possibility that this area is a promising place for encouraging your engagement in love and romance.

Prepare for love and romance

So what's cluttering up the areas of your home that are primed for love and romance? Principally let's start with the south west of your home, the south west of your living room and your bedroom, or any area of your home environment that you choose to dedicate to your personal relationship. Take a good long look at these areas of your home. What can you see there – wonderful photographic images of yourself and your partner, a bunch of red roses, symbols of your love and affection?

Believe us when we tell you that we have encountered some amazingly unhelpful items cluttering up people's romance areas – from general piles of 'stuff', to serene Buddha statues [Buddha was a celibate teacher], objects or photographs belonging to past relationships, spiky plants, bits of dead driftwood, unsuitable pictures eg. a deserted beach, wild horses – one lady even displayed a model of the grim reaper there!

Are the items and décor you currently have in your love and romance areas appropriate? If not, why not? You may feel a smile come over as you go through this process. Truthfully, could you do with a clear out and a spring clean? If so, now is the time to take everything out and start afresh.

Focus Features – placing on purpose – physical reminders

After your cleansing revelation, you can introduce items to your love and romance areas [particularly the south west], to enrich your existing relationship or enhance your chances of meeting someone special. Your Focus Feature placements should be things that have positive, possibly symbolic, meaning for you. Here are some ideas and suggestions, they are not meant to be prescriptive, just do what feels good for you, only one or two things at a time:

- Display a photograph of yourself and your partner happily together.

- Display a symbolic object or image that represents love and romance. Traditionally a pair of mandarin ducks was thought to do the trick but you can try a pair of anything that appeals to you. Or how about something already paired? For example, a small version of Rodin's sculpture 'The Kiss' or a print of Gustav Klimt's picture of the same name. If you are in a relationship, it should be something that you both admire. If you are single, choose something that promotes your ideal view of a loving relationship.

- Place a piece of rose quartz on top of a book of love poems or romantic sayings – periodically read a few to each other.

- Hang a heart shape crystal in a suitable window to catch the sunshine and display beautiful rainbows signifying the potential for love in many colours.

- Fill a vase with gorgeous flowers – red, pink or yellow are particularly symbolic of long-lasting earthy love. There's plenty of choice: roses, peonies, pink carnations, yellow favourite flowers, a pot of geraniums – just ensure they look fresh and always remove dying blooms.

- Decorate your romance area with a passionate colour, possibly a splash of red or pink peach tones but primarily whatever colour feels sensual to you.

- Light a rose scented candle or burn rose incense or your favourite scent.

- If you have written yourself a letter [ACTION A], then place it in one of your romance areas. Alternatively, take a few minutes now to write down your wishes for love and a flourishing relationship. Place your composition in a red envelope in your romance area. You can put the envelope on a beautiful ceramic plate if you like. Always be careful what you wish for!

ACTION C: Your character cue

This is an exercise designed to help you find the best way 'to respond well' in a personal relationship rather than 'to react badly'. It can help you to cut out the critical, complaining, carping communications and replace them with patience, empathy and good humour.

Imagine that you are a character in your own life play and that your surname is Nice or Considerate or Kind or any word that 'does it for you'. Whether you are Mr. Peter Nice or David Serene, Mrs. Lorna Calm or Miss Carol Kind – welcome to the stage of your live performance. In order to remember to act the part of your special character, even when the going gets tough, you adopt 'a character cue'.

Your personal character cue is a potent conditioner for good relationship communications. All you need is a physical object that is always about your person and available to be touched. For this reason, the best items are rings, watches, pendants, talismans, bracelets, amulets etc. You choose a special 'character cue' stone or crystal or chain or material item that you wear or carry with you at all times.

Here's how it works

We all think and behave occasionally in ways that are inappropriate, unkind and sometimes hurtful. We do not like ourselves for this but often, even though we know we are causing an argument or being unreasonable and moody, we just do not seem able to stop the flow. Our emotional selves somehow go into overdrive and we get carried along on the tide of raised voices, aggressive speech, threatening body language or sulky withdrawal.

Your character cue allows you immediately to 'kick in' a third party – your nice self! Touching your cue object, serves as a physical reminder that your character needs a prompt. It is time for your big entrance as Mr, Mrs. or Ms Nice or Calm or whatever you have selected. The more you rehearse and practice with your character cue, the more you are able to show your loving compassionate qualities. This is because you are, in effect, conditioning yourself to the response behaviour of your chosen persona which is also inherently your nice kind considerate self.

When to use

The sort of circumstances where your character cue is particularly useful is when you find yourself feeling annoyed and irritated by your partner or potential partner, if you are dating. See for yourself how using a character cue changes the way you react in such situations. It helps to put things in perspective and bring out your mediation qualities for compromise and peaceful co-existence.

The secret of actually being Mr, Mrs or Ms Nice on a forever basis is to acknowledge the good things you already have together, to improve the things that you can realistically improve and learn to accept and deal with the things that are outside your control to change. Then you can face the world together in harmony.

ACTION D: Make a difference – change something

If you'd like to try something different, we offer a few suggestions which may help you to add something extra for mutual benefit – either [a] within a relationship or [b] if you are looking for a new partner.

[a] Existing relationship choices-for-change

In order to keep your relationship alive and sparkling, one or two variations to your current regime may do the trick.

Personal effort: first you could consider any changes you can work on personally. For example, if you want to learn to be less critical, tell yourself that every time you start to criticise your partner, you will immediately hear it as a cue to re-think, stop and take a deep breath or count to 10, and deflect your criticism to constructive suggestion or a request for help. The time schedule here is immediate! Likewise, if you want to give more time to your relationship – start today. But work out how you can sustain the giving of this extra time, otherwise it will be a one-minute wonder.

An entirely different issue could be that your self-esteem is low, or that you're overly self-conscious and unhappy with your body image, so much so that it is affecting your relationship – body image and self-esteem are covered in the 5th and 9th Enrichments Experience. In particular, the 5th Enrichment includes food, exercise, perception and reality. It allows you to highlight practical ways in which you can start to make best use of your body. It also allows you to look at the way your mind 'sees' your body. These factors all impact your personal relationship.

Partner effort: these are the changes that you would like to see your partner make. Here you need to be extremely diplomatic [and loving!], and try to gain ownership from your partner for the changes. If you are unable to gain consent here, you can accept this is the case for the time being. We suggest you go ahead and start to make your own changes. However, as the whole point of a relationship is that it consists of two people, at some stage you will want to raise these issues with your partner. By setting a good example, he or she is more likely to be open to the idea of change.

Joint effort: together you might agree to initiate changes that require joint effort. This can, to some extent, be a way of overcoming any problems you may encounter when encouraging your partner to make personal changes. For example, you may be squeaky clean yourself but feel your partner's personal hygiene leaves much to be desired. Although this is your partner's problem, it impacts on your life. So you could devise a system where every time you, or your partner, are ready to make love, you introduce bathing or showering as part of the intimacy.

In the same way, if there is a significant difference in your approach to earning, saving or spending money which is causing disagreement, then try to work out and agree what you both feel is 'reasonable and sensible' within your particular income stream and budget constraints.

What about your respective emotional needs? Both men and women have a deep-rooted emotional requirement for love and affection – are you both aware of each other's needs in this regard? Can you talk openly about these needs and how you can show appreciation for each other? Discuss and work through any areas or problems that require joint change. If your partner is unwilling to participate in this, then you need to ask yourself 'why?'.

At the end of the day, you and your partner are the only people who can actually bring into being the kind of relationship you both desire. With honest openness you can succeed – over to you – and remember that wrapping your requests up in a humorous package often works wonders.

Major relationship change: if you are experiencing serious difficulties in your relationship requiring fundamental change, then you may want to get some outside help. Professional advice is best used as early as possible if there is to be a good chance of reconciliation or successful mediation. Never underestimate the pain, guilt and anger associated with the break-up of a close relationship – reconciliation is sometimes a good option. Remember you both chose to get together at one time – are the good reasons for being together still there beneath the discord?

If you are considering leaving your relationship, particularly if there are children involved, then set some quiet time aside to project forward and examine the realities of a break up. Write down the plus and minus points in terms of your residential and financial situation, and also how you see yourself, and your dependents, coping mentally and emotionally.

Make sure you are aware of, and equipped to cope with, the damaging feelings that often surface at the time of a partnership break up. Even if you feel that the break up is inevitable and is primarily 'not your fault', you will probably have days when you are awash with anguish – be prepared to stand by your choices and ask your friends for support. We wish you good luck, good planning and a fresh future.

[b] New relationship choices-for-change

As you are no doubt aware, there are many self-help books and magazine articles on meeting a new partner and maintaining a relationship thereafter, so your next stop may be the local bookstore or online retailer.

Best of all be brave – get right out there and join a club, check in for night school, take up a new sport, sing in a choir, invite your friends round for a meal, organise a trip to the theatre/cinema, register with an on-line dating site, volunteer for charity work, take a weekend 'activity' break, attend seminars and conferences relating to your work or hobbies, book a singles holiday, join a local meetup group [www.meetup.com] – a brilliant organisation for bringing people together in your area to share in a wide variety of interests – pop in your post code and see what's on offer.

The secret is not to do any of these activities with the sole objective of meeting a partner, but to do them for their own sake, enjoy the experience and live a little. It is often when you are not looking that someone appears.

And remember 'you never get a second chance to make a good first impression', so be responsible for looking your best at all times – take care of your mental and physical welfare. Your charisma will instantly shine through if you walk tall and smile – it is a guaranteed 'turn on' for the opposite sex – try it and find out.

Love well – give and receive

Whatever you decide to do, make sure it is in tune with the essence of the 2nd Enrichment – to be a happy loving person either in your existing relationship or ready to find a life partner or content to be single and use your time in other ways. To give and to receive love is one of the highest human undertakings and there's an inspiring Greek proverb to motivate us: *"The heart that loves is always young".*

THE 3rd ENRICHMENT EXPERIENCE

Life-long learning; curiosity; engaging new ideas; personal growth; respect for parents, ancestors, elders, teachers, coaches and leaders; initiation and germination; discovery. *"Learning and rejoicing go hand in hand"* Epicurus.

The 3rd Enrichment Experience teaches us always to be curious – amazing vitality can be ours when we embrace new things. Here is an opportunity to explore our incredible ability to learn – to memorise, to accumulate facts and figures, to appreciate the wonders of nature, to enjoy the miracle of language and the written word, to pluck an idea out of thin air and cultivate it, to be fresh and exciting, to broaden the mind over many years. As Epictetus remarked *"spirited curiosity is an emblem of the flourishing life"*.

Interested and interesting

Making a conscious effort to be interested in all sorts of things going on in the world around you [that's a lot of things!], will ensure that your life is permanently interesting. It will enable you to take advantage of opportunities for furthering your knowledge and skills, and give you more confidence in social conversational situations.

Whatever their age, people who appear younger than they actually are, invariably have that 'added spark' – the charisma that comes from keeping the mind fresh and active. They are always pushing the boundaries and being bored or boring is not an option. By participating in the 3rd Enrichment, you can engage this youthful aspect of learning and appreciate that variety is indeed 'the spice of life'.

Researchers who study ways to combat dementia in later life recommend keeping your brain as active as possible post-retirement by doing word and number puzzles, playing games such as bridge, chess or scrabble, reading books, watching educational programmes and always being open to learning new things. However we can all engage in these mind-stretching activities whatever our age.

Ignore the maxim 'you can't teach an old dog new tricks' – it is only true if we are talking about things like learning a musical instrument in later life to world-class performance level, or learning Olympic-style gymnastics when we are past the first flush of youth. These extreme examples aside, life-long learning is the most wonderful gift that we can give ourselves. And today there are so many opportunities that the greatest problem we face is deciding what to do first. What would you like to do first?

Showing your admiration

Another aspect of the 3rd Enrichment is the chance to show respect for the people who give their time to help us learn new things and develop our skill set. This includes formal educators such as school and college teachers, alongside youth workers, sports coaches, music tutors and, of course, parents and carers.

Do you feel respect for all the people who help you to learn? Are you grateful for their dedication and effort? Can you appreciate that it isn't always an easy job for them? There is great merit in paying the occasional compliment to show that you really value what their tuition and care has meant for your life. The Buddha wisely said, *"In one's family, respect and listening are the source of harmony"*.

Sometimes we even learn important lessons from our interactions with the people who 'press our buttons', and from our own 'mis-takes'. Are you able to see any of these learning opportunities in your life right now?

Even if you rarely see one or other of your parents, that person is still your parent. Whether your relationship is a good quality one or a poor quality one, it will have a subtle impact on your life. It is healthy to acknowledge and accept parental relationships, however they manifest, and be clear as to how they influence your choices and decisions, if at all.

Then there are the role models whom you can admire and strive to emulate. They may be courageous friends or relatives, charity workers, philanthropists, sporting stars, artists, writers, singers, actors, broadcasters, politicians or small children who show you how to smile – anyone whose life influences you in a positive way.

Talking history

As you think about the 3rd Enrichment, we also encourage you to honour your elders and ancestors – those who came before you in the family, whose lives were necessary in order for you to be born. Talking to your elderly grandparents about their early experiences and their recollections of their own parents and grandparents, gives them an enjoyable trip down memory lane while you gain a fascinating link with your own history. The current trend for researching family trees and organising reunions that include distant family members is very much in the spirit of the 3rd Enrichment.

The 3rd Enrichment Experience Action Area

The following ideas may help you discover what, if anything, you could change in your routine to enhance opportunities for learning, showing respect for teachers, coaches and elders, and re-engaging with your youthful persona when curiosity was a key feature of everyday life. Choose the actions that resonate with you, disregard the others.

ACTION A: Questions & answers – your motivating letter

Write yourself a personal letter [Dear Me . . . and the date] in which you answer one or more of the following questions:

Thinking about your opportunities for learning new things, do you feel you are taking advantage of them? Are you still curious about life in general – most 3 year olds constantly ask 'why' about almost everything? Do you have a particular interest of which you are keen to expand your knowledge?

Whatever your age, is there anything obvious you could do right now to give yourself the opportunity to learn something new or to increase your knowledge and skills in an existing field of interest? Over the next 3-5 years?

Are you appreciative of, and able to compliment, your family members and teachers who give up their time to help you progress? Do you take an interest in your ancestral heritage? Do you have role models who inspire you?

As you write your letter, you may be inspired to highlight areas where you could develop your skills and interests, and possibly spend more time with people from whom you can learn or with whom you can share new experiences? Maybe write a couple of sentences about how you intend to develop your immense capacity for life-long learning from now on. If necessary, make a definite plan to attend classes or spend time with the appropriate teachers or relatives.

Likewise, be realistic about your relationships with parents and grandparents and find ways to make them as nurturing as possible for all concerned. Are there any obvious pointers as to where you could realistically start to initiate choices-for-change? Be constructive so that your letter expresses your positive intentions. You can add to it anytime.

Headline your final paragraph with the words "Glad to be alive." Now choose three things, related in some way to the 3rd Enrichment, that 'make your heart sing'. How about the amazing ability you have to learn or the admiration and respect you feel for your teachers or relatives? Or possibly you can see the promise of something new. An easy way to do this is to finish the sentence: "I'm glad that I ...."

Put your letter in an envelope [preferably green] and place it in the east of your home or study area if you have one. The significance of this will become apparent in ACTION B.

ACTION B: Create an inspiring environment

Take a look around your home and see where the learning and respect areas are? Where do you feel most comfortable thinking, reading, writing or generally digesting new material? Where do you watch or listen to educational programmes or take in current affairs? Where do you soak up inspirational music? Where do you display photographs of your parents and grandparents? Which areas in your home do you think your ancestors might empathise with?

Although the places we associate with learning – schools, colleges, universities, career enhancement centres, contemplative retreats – are mighty important, perhaps it is in our own homes that much of our true learning takes place. And while we consider anywhere in the home worthy of a learning experience, we would like to highlight the eastern aspect of your property.

The east is symbolic of sunrise – a new dawn every day, a fresh start, the awakening morning light, the growth potential of springtime, the germinating seed, new wood and green foliage, fulfilling relationships with parents and teachers. All these images can help you to decide how you want to organise and decorate the eastern areas of your home or any other areas where you feel 'refreshment' is called for.

Spring clean yourself and the east of your home

'Spring clean' is the operative phrase for the 3rd Enrichment. This time it is to 'spring clean' your life. What is cluttering up your learning and respect areas? Have a look around and you will know intuitively where you need to have a clear out and a clean-up. The best way is to remove every single item from the areas you have identified and then replace – beautifully – only those which serve your purpose for the next phase of learning and respect. Question what is helpful and what is hindering – which objects, fixtures, fittings, colours and materials inspire you?

Focus Features – placing on purpose – physical reminders

Once you have finished your 'spring clean', you can install some physical Habitat Affect reminders. Introduce Focus Features that will stimulate your learning opportunities – whatever you choose it will be personal to you – no-one else can tell you the best placements. Similarly, if you feel so minded, display an item or two honouring senior members of your family, teachers and role models.

Here are some suggestions for the east of your home or the particular areas you have identified as being conducive to learning and heritage – only do what feels good for you.

- Display photographs of your parents, grandparents and helpful teachers.
- Display a photograph of your high school or college graduation.
- Organise furniture or shelving for books and digital devices of educational value.
- Place a vigorous pot plant in appropriate natural light and keep it well watered.
- Grow some herbs on an eastern windowsill.
- Use the colour green for decorative purposes.
- Brainstorm yourself and hatch out new ideas in the east of your home.
- Make notes about your ideas and learning aspirations and display them on a notice board/magnetic surface or write them on a whiteboard/blackboard – keep them fresh and updated.
- Enjoy the glorious view of sunrise – new beginnings – from an east window.
- Hang a bamboo wind chime in the east and be inspired by its mellow tones.
- Write down your wishes for learning something new on a piece of green paper, fold it in half and place it in an attractive wooden bowl. Re-visit frequently and update with whatever it is you intend to learn next!

ACTION C: What and when to learn – how to make it happen

This is an ideal planning exercise if you are the sort of person who likes an organised systematic approach to engaging your mind in new things.

Take a sheet of paper landscape and rule 2 vertical lines so that you end up with three equal columns.

[1] Head the first column 'What I want to learn'. Underneath write down anything and everything about which you would like to know more. From learning a foreign language to woodwork or car mechanics, researching a potential holiday destination or revisiting history lessons, finding out what goes on inside plants, trying to get to grips with algebra, compiling your family tree, taking bridge lessons – it's your list so it can be as diverse as you like.

[2] Head the second column 'When I will do this'. Opposite each item in the first column, write a timeline for your potential learning experience. For instance, you could do a 10 week adult learning class [or whatever is on offer locally] in the autumn term or you could specify a period of say 3 months in which to read as much as possible about your chosen subject – the way you decide your timeline is entirely individual. Learning to ski for example usually requires seasonal access to snow.

Because there will probably be far too many things in the first column to do all at once, you will need to set priorities – you could choose to learn something in the more distant future but it still makes sense to think about it now.

[3] Head the third column 'How I will make it happen'. This is your task bar – the things you need to put into your schedule so that your intentions become reality. An example would be to book an activity or cultural holiday well in advance or sign up for classes or visit the library twice a week etc. Your priorities in the second column will, to a certain extent, dictate how specific you are in detailing the required tasks to 'make it happen'. Leave room at the end of the column for a big tick when you have accomplished your learning mission!

The idea of this exercise is to make learning something you 'do on purpose' but also 'do for pleasure'. If it becomes a chore, then the object of the exercise will not have been achieved. So you might think of this as light-hearted learning entertainment with some very real and rewarding benefits.

ACTION D: Make a difference – change something

This is your chance to make a commitment to change something for the better. You could set yourself some definite learning challenges and monitor your progress. You could keep a daily/weekly journal which might include your interactions with people from whom you learn and mention specific ways of showing your respect. You could commit to being fully alive – forever – to all opportunities for learning and respect which are constantly arising within your realm.

Learning invigorates healthy minds

Whatever you decide to do, make sure it is in tune with the essence of the 3rd Enrichment – that is to inspire your curiosity, enhance your experience of learning new things, to show respect for those who have gone before you and for the people of culture and skill who educate you – all of which helps to keep your life fresh and interesting.

THE 4th ENRICHMENT EXPERIENCE

Fortunate blessings; abundance; prosperity; wealth; money; financial planning; budgeting; knowing what is enough for one's needs; generosity and altruism. *"Contentment is freedom – count your blessings."* Anon.

The 4th Enrichment Experience is both challenging and rewarding – it tackles an area of our lives that we tend to keep hidden, but which has a massive impact on how we conduct ourselves on a daily basis. Yes – we are talking about money – our financial well-being or the lack of it.

We are also checking out the way we feel about 'having enough' and 'being fortunate' – which do not absolutely depend on the amount of money we have in the bank or invested in shares or property. In this context, we start with a few words on 'needs versus wants'. NB. If you are heavily in debt or just extremely anxious about your financial situation, we recommend you seek professional help.

Your 'needs' may really be 'wants'

In order to develop a practical framework for attracting good fortune, it is wise to assess your essential 'needs' as opposed to your luxury 'wants'. Whatever your particular needs, and the state of your personal finances, this is a chance for you to take a step aside and see if there are ways in which you could improve your current monetary situation or possibly just your attitude towards it.

If you choose to take up the challenge, you can differentiate your true needs from your wants and desires. The latter represent your attachment to all sorts of things that are not essential for a healthy happy life. Krishnamurti summed this up explicitly by saying *"when you desire, you become the slave to that object of desire."* One 'need' we could do well to adopt is the need to acquire resistance against insidious commercial propaganda aimed at increasing our desire for more stuff – we must learn to be disciplined consumers.

Today, many of us have built up complex lifestyles based on 'perceived needs', some of which are unnecessary and may be socially or media driven. For example, designer labels, state-of-the-art entertainment equipment, second homes, membership of clubs we rarely attend, expensive creams we rarely use, jewellery we are frightened of losing, computer games we never play etc. At the other end of the scale are those of us who are living hand to mouth and wondering how to manage debts that may be spiralling out of control.

Low cost contentment

The good news is that our financial circumstances can improve significantly simply by identifying the things we really need in order to cultivate contentment. For instance, walking or running in the fresh air is free, expensive gym membership maybe just that – expensive. We can restyle out-of-date clothes, learn how to put up shelves and renovate old furniture, stop buying unhealthy sweets and sugary fizzy drinks, organise 'pot luck' suppers with friends, 'eat in' pretending home is a restaurant, make personalised greetings cards, listen to radio news and read library books rather than buying magazines and newspapers – the list can be as long and diverse as your imagination allows.

Another piece of useful advice comes from the novelist Julian Barnes: *"You should never make the mistake of comparing the inside of one's own life with the outside of someone else's."* Wise words when it comes to wrestling with the green-eyed monsters of jealousy and envy. These tainted traits are often lodged subconsciously in our minds and need to be acknowledged in order to be overcome. Both are arch enemies of contentment which is important for our financial well-being.

Contentment, rather than lazy complacency, is happiness and satisfaction with the life we are living in combination with an appreciation of our potential to develop further. Whether comfortably off, just about solvent or financially struggling, we can all benefit from learning to live more simply and contentedly in an increasingly complex world.

The 4th Enrichment Experience Action Area

You may like to engage with all or some of the following suggestions to help you decide what, if anything, you might do differently with regard to your finances. The aim is for you to understand your relationship with money and your feelings about 'needs' and 'wants', budgeting, encouraging good fortune and being satisfied with your lot. Knowing more about what makes you tick financially will enable you to identify any choices-for-change so you can celebrate the 4th Enrichment with gratitude and contentment. Choose the actions that resonate with you, disregard the others.

ACTION A: Questions & answers – your motivating letter

Write yourself a personal letter [Dear Me . . . and the date] in which you answer one or more of the following questions:

What is your general attitude towards money – do you work hard to earn it, save it whenever possible and live within your means or are you spending more than you earn, using your credit card too liberally or resorting to personal loans?

Thinking about your personal finances, do you have any current issues you can identify? Are you good at budgeting?

Do you have any dependents? If so, how does your responsibility for them impact your financial position?

As you write your letter, you may find other questions arising that are specific to your current finances, in which case include answers to these as well. Have any of your answers highlighted areas where you could realistically start to initiate some changes? Maybe write a couple of sentences about how you could develop different coping strategies for dealing with the inflow and outflow of money – you can always add to this later. Try to avoid negativity – your letter can be an expression of positive intentions.

Headline your final paragraph with the words "Glad to be alive." Now choose three things, related in some way to the 4th Enrichment, that 'make your heart sing'. They might be to do with having your finances well organised, contentment with having your true needs met, giving yourself permission to have a treat because 'you're worth it' or celebrating the fact that your generosity has enabled someone less fortunate to benefit in some way. An easy way to do this is to finish the sentence: "I'm glad that ...."

Now put your completed letter in an envelope [preferably green or red] and place it in the south east of your home or the south east of the area where you deal with finances. The significance of this will become apparent in ACTION B.

ACTION B: Create an inspiring environment

In ancient oriental society, having a house located in an auspicious physical environment with a beautiful entrance was considered essential for the wealth and prosperity of the household. While most of us today are not in the financial position to choose an amazing external location, we can make every effort to keep our homes neat and attractive both inside and out.

The traditional Feng Shui view is that handsome uncluttered surroundings enhance opportunities for 'money luck', with the south east of the property being known as the wealth area. This can refer to a south eastern room, or the south east of your living room or the south east of the area where you handle your finances. Compass directions aside, your chances of prosperity and good fortune are greatly improved if you always strive to be sensible in your financial and altruistic actions, wherever they take place.

Clearing and organising – develop an easy-to-use system

Let's start with how you keep all the papers, files, bills, bank statements, e-docs etc. associated with your household and personal finances. Be honest, is your system a good one? Does everything 'have a home' within the system. Do you have easy-to-use files stored on attractive shelving or neatly in a cupboard or suitably kept in appropriate folders on your computer? If you use a desk, table or telephone for monetary reasons, are they well-appointed? When new paperwork or e-files connected to your finances arrive, do you deal with them appropriately or allow them to stack up and get into a muddle?

Now is an opportunity to clean up your act – both your physical storage space and the system for storing financially-related information on your computer. Spend some time thinking about what would work best for you and your family, then get clearing and re-organising.

A visit to an office supply stores may be necessary [box files are really useful]. How about some new shelving? What would be a good system for storing information on your computer so that it is quick to retrieve – plus back it up on encrypted cloud storage, a memory stick or other e-device.

A bit eccentric but please check for leaks

The next question, somewhat strangely, is: do you have any water leaks on your property – a dripping tap perhaps, a cracked pipe, a faulty ballcock, seepage from a septic tank? If so, please get it fixed immediately – this is a symbolic sign that your money may be flowing out of the house! As for your cloakroom and bathroom – please ensure that the loo seat is always replaced after use and the door closed. OK this may sound wacky but, bear with us, it just might work.

Focus Features – placing on purpose – physical reminders

Apart from a general tidy up, there are certain Focus Feature placements – summarised below – deemed to be helpful for your financial welfare and general good fortune. These physical reminders of your intent to manage your monetary affairs to the very best of your ability can serve as token prompts if you find yourself getting off track.

- Symbolise your chances of monetary good fortune and growing prosperity by placing a jade plant [also known as a money plant or friendship plant] in the south east of your home or in the area where you do your finances, provided there is plenty of natural daylight. Money plants thrive in sunshine and are very easy to propagate – hopefully like your finances.

- If you want to revitalise your wealth area – the south eastern aspect of your property – consider a splash of lime green on a wall or as an accessory. The wealth area is associated with the element 'wood', so anything representing wood or water [glass items for instance], which feeds wood, is considered auspicious.

- Take a beautiful wooden bowl and fill it with something that makes you think of abundance – whatever represents good fortune for you – coins, shells, a precious stone, rice or another non-perishable food. Refresh it often.

- Alternatively take a beautiful wooden bowl and leave it unfilled to remind you that the empty vessel is ready to receive or put an inspirational saying in it as an aide-mémoire. Set aside a few minutes to contemplate these words and count your blessings, such as they are already. If you have written yourself a letter [as detailed in ACTION A], you can also put it in this bowl.

- Write a list of your financial and altruistic wishes, put it in a green or red envelope and place in the south east or in the area of your home where you have decided to honour the 4th Enrichment. When you give money to a deserving cause, you will often find it is soon replaced by an unexpected windfall – however small – take note.

- If you are prepared to spend time looking after live fish, then an aquarium placed in the south east is considered good luck. A water feature will also do the trick – ensure the water is flowing towards you. However, this requires electricity at a time when we are trying to cut down on energy use so it is not a preferred option.

- If the south eastern aspect of your garden falls away too steeply, plant a robust shrub/tree or place a solid feature or retaining fence there.

ACTION C: The 'money mind map' exercise

Making a mind map about your relationship with money helps you to enter a 'climate of consent' for thinking about your finances in a different way. This is your chance to have an 'out of the box' experience and hopefully gain a few insights that weren't obvious before.

Start with two sheets of blank unlined paper. Get into a comfortable position that allows you to draw and write easily. Take the first sheet of paper and place a smallish circle in the middle with the word 'money' written inside it.

Now close your eyes and breathe in deeply to the count of 7, hold for a moment or two and then breathe out to the count of 7. Repeat this 'counting' breathing a few times until you feel nice and relaxed.

Open your eyes, continue with the steady breathing without counting, and think about the word 'money' sitting in the middle of your piece of paper. Try to imagine yourself in various situations as appropriate to you, for example:

- earning money
- handling money
- being in a bank or online banking
- investing money
- buying something you really need
- buying something you don't really need
- browsing online stores
- gambling online
- giving someone you love an expensive present
- giving a present because it's expected of you

- giving to a charity you care passionately about
- giving to a charity because of social pressure to do so
- feeling anxious and worried about money
- feeling contentment around money
- feeling that you have enough for 'a good life'

Now write down all the words or phrases you can possibly think of that you associate with money and the state of your finances. Do this in a random fashion all over the sheet of paper. Don't worry if it looks a mess, the idea is to free yourself from the normal constraints of orderly lists so that all the issues, however amazing, are on the piece of paper. Take as long as you like and feel free to repeat similar ideas using different words – just write them down as they come into your head.

When you have finished scribbling, put your pen down and take a long hard look at all those words. Choose some of the words or phrases as your 'primary triggers' that can be directly linked with the central money circle. Draw a circle around each of these words or phrases with a coloured pen and then draw lines to link them to the money circle.

In the same way, other words or phrases may be linked to the primary triggers – these are 'secondary triggers' – draw coloured lines between the secondary triggers and the primary triggers which they link with [a secondary trigger may link with more than one primary trigger].

You may now find that there are a few words or phrases that you want to discard, so cross them out. And, of course, you may want to add a few more words as you go along.

What you are looking at now is probably a complete mishmash of words and lines. Nonetheless, it contains the core ingredients of your current relationship with money. So the next step is to tidy it up.

Take the second sheet of paper and re-draw your mind map starting with the 'money' circle in the middle but with the primary and secondary triggers rearranged, so that the map is easier to read and understand.

Now have a really good look at what you have created and the possible financial scenarios that are either holding you back or offering you great opportunities.

Any insights staring you in the face? You may be able to see, and accept, changes in your attitude towards money plus practical things you can do to achieve a sense of financial balance. If this is the case, write three sentences across the bottom of your map stating your intentions for the short, medium and long-term.

ACTION D: Make a difference – change something

This is your chance to commit to doing something differently in the way you handle your finances. You can choose a motivating goal and the steps you need to take to get there. Write a few words about your goal and the specific tasks you intend to do with an achievable time schedule.

Place your composition in the south east of your home or workplace. Whatever you decide to do, make sure it is in tune with the essence of the 4th Enrichment – that is to manage your finances responsibly, to acknowledge the difference between needs and wants, to enjoy and share whatever fortunate blessings come your way.

THE 5th ENRICHMENT EXPERIENCE

Physical health – your body, food, drink, exercise, sleep, stress; mental and emotional well-being; whole life harmony; finding a balance; equanimity; honesty and responsibility. William Blake captured the essence of the 5th Enrichment Experience when he wrote *"Energy is eternal delight"*.

How often do you experience the tremendous sense of energetic well-being which arises when you are truly healthy in mind and body? The 5th Enrichment is primed to help you realise this glorious feeling which involves every aspect of your life. So, in a very real way, the other 8 enrichments all contribute towards this one and vice-versa.

We maintain that our mental health is totally intertwined with our physicality, so the 5th Enrichment opens with an appreciation of our amazing bodies. We invite you, whatever your shape, size, weight, age or state of health, to take a loving journey through yourself 'appreciating the miracle of me' which you will find in Appendix G. Although simplistic, this 'journey through myself' offers several clues to the secret of good physical and mental health which is what the 5th Enrichment Experience is all about.

Harnessing your power to improve your health

If you are reading this, perhaps your intention is to improve your health by altering some of your existing habits and choosing a different pattern of actions. The 5th Enrichment Experience offers you this 're-creational' opportunity – take from it what you will – remember it is your choice.

Maybe you have a weight issue? Or do you dislike the way 'you think' you look? Are you drinking too much alcohol? Are you a couch potato? Do you 'suffer' from low self-esteem? Feel like you are on an emotional rollercoaster? Are you having trouble sleeping? Maybe there's nothing much 'wrong' but you feel the need to perk up your energy levels?

Just a note about mental health – herein we explore thought, memory and emotions within the typical range. If you have serious mental health issues, then please seek professional medical help.

The ongoing journey is the goal

Ideally we view 'the goal' of good physical and mental health as an uplifting journey – a journey we try to undertake with enthusiasm throughout our lives. Cherishing your health means being responsible for making 'best use' of your mind and body most of the time, while allowing for the occasional lapse without beating yourself up over it. This is not a one-off effort but an ongoing lifetime passage which requires attention and positive intention on a daily basis.

Unfortunately it is all too easy to neglect our physical and mental health completely until we get a stark warning when something goes wrong. Even if we are aware of the importance of good health, we may still think of it as something we 'should' or 'ought' to tackle. Often when there is the idea of 'should' or 'ought', any 'problems' just seem to be insurmountable, so we bury them away and pretend we are quite happy with things the way they are. We may even play the victim and blame other people or our circumstances or our age and stage – anything but make a few changes.

Thinking of your health as an ongoing journey means you can drop the stories and excuses and simply start the journey today – right here, right now. What's stopping you taking that first step, then another and another? One way to get started on the journey is quite simply to change the emphasis of your thinking.

Re-tune your thoughts about health issues

Here are a few examples of how to turn your thoughts or speech around into sensible constructive intentions:

"I'm tired all the time" can become "I'm willing to find ways to feel full of energy";

"I'm overweight" can become "I'm willing to respect my body and enjoy feeding it healthy nourishing food and drink";

"I'm shy and introverted" can become "I'm willing to take a risk in a social situation and see what happens";

"I'm a couch potato" can become "I'm really looking forward to energising my body and mind with an exercise plan that includes brisk walking and other pursuits, something I can stick to without it being a drag";

"I drink too much" can become "I enjoy an alcoholic drink or two but I always eat something first and have a glass of water on the go at the same time, and I know when to stop";

"I'm stressed out with money worries so I fantasise everyday about winning the lottery" can become "I'm a realist about my financial situation so I apply common sense to handling money – the occasional flutter on the lottery is just for fun with no expectations whatsoever".

Be a healthy eater

Using the power of 'thought re-tuning', let's briefly look at the issue of weight loss. Rather than think: "I'm overweight so I'll have to go on a diet [again]", what you intend can be phrased entirely differently: "I want to have an attractive healthy weight body so, every day, I'll treat myself to healthy nourishing foods and keep physically toned by exercising".

Here the accent is on learning to enjoy healthy nourishing food and energy-promoting exercise as a way of creating a healthy body. And, in your heart of hearts, you probably know which foods and exercises are good for your health, rather than a slimming diet of another's prescription.

In fact, we maintain that some rigid diet approaches can be counter-productive, leading to yo-yo dieting. For example, dieters who restrict food intake by counting calories over a long period, have the daily task of working out what they can and cannot eat. This constant focus on food is itself mentally unhealthy and may encourage secret binge eating.

Treating your body with respect and learning to enjoy eating – something you have to do to live – is entirely possible, once you change your attitude towards your physicality. However, we emphasise that not all poor relationships with food have similar roots. Tragically, for some, disordered eating and poor body image are present time manifestations of serious psychological trauma encountered in the past. Although the same healthy eating and exercise approach is applicable, if you are affected in this way, you should consult a qualified professional for appropriate help. Issues around food are covered in some detail later in this chapter.

Be a non-smoker

Try the same thought re-tuning logic with trying to quit smoking. This is a notorious example of an activity that does not succeed unless the person concerned really wants to stop smoking. Here the accepted goal is "I am going to be a non-smoker" or even "I am a non-smoker" which is different from saying "I want to stop smoking".

You can visualise yourself as a non-smoker and all the benefits that accrue to this state. This is entirely different from 'wanting to stop smoking' and then trying 'to start to stop'. Here you are focusing on a theoretical want rather than the definite state of being a non-smoker. However, nicotine is a powerful drug and allowances are to be made for its addictive qualities – more of this later.

Responsibility for personal choices

The 5th Enrichment requires you to be entirely truthful about your health habits – excellent, acceptable but in need of a makeover, or complete overhaul required? In his book 'The End of Illness' Dr David B Agus says "... *make it your goal to take full responsibility for your health every single day no matter what life throws at you.*"

It is within your power to choose to live more healthily in ways that are both achievable, allowing for a certain degree of effort, and sustainable – for the rest of your life. Gradually you will notice the path of good health getting easier as you feel more confident about yourself and you may even become energetically able to help others follow your lead.

Have a clear vision of your health needs

Getting to grips with your health issues can be disturbing at first because it requires complete honesty and you may not always like what you see. However, if you approach your physical and mental health within a boundary of self-respect, and take responsibility for working out the practical things you can actually do, life will instantly start to feel different. You are the only person capable of doing this for you.

If you are open to trying this approach, you could start by making a raw statement about yourself as things stand right now. We say 'raw' because it may be uncomfortable for you to 'tell it like it is' and what comes out may be somewhat negative. If this is the case, the next step is to move from your negative-type statement to something you can work with in a positive frame of mind.

To do this, it helps to have a clear vision of what you really need for good health. Without this vision, any change or 'solution' is less likely to be wholeheartedly embraced by your mental controller – which of course is you. By making a personal promise to achieve the best health possible for your particular body and mind throughout your ongoing life journey – you are likely to succeed.

The 5th Enrichment Experience Action Area

Physical and mental health is, of course, an immensely complex subject so we can only touch on the more obvious areas. The aim is to help you to think deeply, and possibly differently, about your health so that 'your common-sense' prevails, helping you achieve vitality and wellness most of the time. To this end, you can choose to engage with some of the following suggestions designed to help you decide what, if anything, you might be up for changing. Feel free to pick 'n' mix as appropriate to your personal situation.

ACTION A: Questions & answers – your motivating letter

First read about the various health issues below – body image; relationship with food; smoking; alcohol; exercise; sleeping; cleansing; stress – and decide which, if any, you would like to explore in more detail.

If you like, write yourself a personal health letter [Dear Me …… and the date] in which you answer the questions about each health issue as appropriate to your specific situation.

A1: Your general body image

Your body image is the mental picture you have of your physical form. Image is not fact; it is often the result of biased assumptions. You may be a fashion model size, or a lean and muscular athletic type, but still be worried by your appearance. You may be a robust female or a skinny male and be very happy in your body.

The actual fact of physical form is often not what counts to someone who doesn't like their body or specific parts of it. Harbouring irrational views about aspects of the body [body dysmorphia] is a surprisingly common issue, particularly for young adults with the presumed pressure to look like an airbrushed celebrity, a computer-generated model or to be seen as popular – 'liked' – on social networking sites.

Your wisdom on this subject comes from understanding that appreciation of your physical body is a mental health issue. The actual physical appearance of your body is not necessarily the same as the body image that you hold in your mind. And your mind's view can dictate what 'you see' in the mirror. Unfortunately, as already mentioned, there is a tendency today for people to compare themselves not just with their friends but also with high maintenance ultra-styled superstars. Perhaps take a moment to think if you are someone who is influenced in this way?

So is healthy body image all down to your personal choice of how you decide to think? Not quite, because your actual body may, in fact, be unhealthy. Having a healthy image of an unhealthy physical body might also be an issue for some. We need to bring the reality in line with the perception and vice-versa. For those of you wanting to improve your health, developing a healthy body image is an essential part of the 'creating change' process.

Question yourself about your body image

If you feel you have an issue with regard to your body image, what exactly is it? Write your answer in your health letter to yourself. Try to add some thoughts on how to deal with this in a practical sustainable way.

Think about what your answer reveals and start to see yourself in a new light. Whatever your body type, if you pay attention to your deportment – 'walk tall' – dress to flatter your shape and project a happy persona, you will automatically look, and feel, better. And always remember 'the most attractive thing you can wear is a smile'.

A2: Your relationship with food

Some 2400 years ago Hippocrates wrote: *"Let your food be your treatment, and your treatment be your food."* Similarly, in traditional Indian culture, Ayurvedic medicine starts with what you eat. You have to eat to live. Whatever your actual weight or perceived body image, a relationship with food is unavoidable. You can decide to make it a good relationship or a poor relationship. You can choose to understand the difference between an unhealthy eating pattern involving denial, addiction or even self-loathing, or an enjoyable appreciation of life-sustaining nourishment.

NB: If you are exhibiting signs of anorexia or bulimia nervosa please see your doctor. The suggestions herein are not a substitute for help with these serious conditions.

You are what you eat – so choose your foods wisely

The most important tool in your mental store cupboard is your practical common sense. If in doubt about the value of a particular food, then trust your intuition – it is that simple. Deep down you will know if something is wholesome and nourishing or if it is just a mass of 'empty' calories disguised by a clever food manufacturer as an irresistible tasty treat.

Your body deserves only the best – and that does not necessarily mean the most expensive. If, for example, you choose wholemeal bread and pasta, rather than the goodness-stripped 'white' varieties, you will feel full sooner, so you will need to eat less. This means far better nutrition for an equivalent cost and fewer calories.

Treating yourself as a rubbish bin for artificially produced foods packaged as mouth-watering must-haves is really quite dangerous for your long term health. In the short term, you may well experience 'a high' after consuming some sugar-laden fatty delicacy, followed by a lethargic low, and so the cycle repeats itself.

Many people are feeling tired these days due in part to a poor quality diet. In Appendix H we have listed some foods that boost your energy level – not just as a five minute wonder – plus a list of foods that deplete well-being after an initial unsustainable surge. If you want to go into the subject in more depth, there are numerous books and websites devoted to nutrition and health. Find the medium that suits you and add zest to your life by eating for health.

If you want to lose weight show respect for your body

Respect for your body will naturally lead you to want the best for it. We repeat: why use your body as a dustbin for too much food? Why gobble up highly processed 'artificial' foods that bear little resemblance to the foods your body has evolved to thrive on? You like the taste and texture? Our food manufacturers certainly make sure that 'engineered' food products taste absolutely gorgeous – that's their trap.

Wouldn't you rather acquire a love for the taste and texture of foods that help give you good health and a contented feeling about your body? How wonderful to be able to choose 'good' food as a friend, and still enjoy the occasional ice-cream or pudding, without being tortured by cravings. It is possible to do this with a change of thinking – developing an understanding of what eating is really all about for you.

Research has shown that the act of keeping a food diary can significantly improve weight loss. We suggest that if the idea of keeping a diary appeals to you, then make it a 'body-respect diary' rather than a food diary. This allows you to take the focus away from food [and the negative aspects of over-concentrating your thinking just on food], to the positive recording of how you are feeling about your newly-emerging body as it starts to take shape.

A word about doing without calorie counting

Counting calories is a popular way that some people use to try to lose weight – and we acknowledge that if this is your preference and it works for you, then fine. However, as we mentioned previously, a daily routine based around counting calories involves quite a lot of time thinking about food and calories, even if you use an online food diary service.

Such thinking can quite easily become obsessive, quite apart from the fact that it forces you to be thinking about food at the expense of thinking about other more worthwhile things. How much better, and eventually less demanding on your thinking time, to educate yourself with information about the basic natural food groups – what is good and healthy and what is not [Appendix H for a start].

Happily, you will be pleased to find there is a magnificent variety of foods you can enjoy, and in reasonable quantity. Often the less processed carbohydrates and lower fat foods are naturally bulkier than highly processed products, so you can fill your plate and feast your eyes.

And plant proteins – fruits and vegetables – are brilliant for adding bulk, with a splash of colour, to any meal.

The idea is to create a super-healthy interest in the enjoyment of buying, preparing and eating food. This approach will feel completely different from negative restrictive diet regimes so many of us have tried in the past.

Talk to yourself in the mirror

"Everything I put in my mouth from now on is something that I have chosen to eat. Mostly I will be eating food as a health-giving experience. Occasionally I may choose to sample foods that are high in fat and processed carbohydrate. I will accept that 'all things in moderation' applies to food as well as to life in general. However, I will no longer view unhealthy foods as 'treats'. Rather my treats will be enjoying a variety of nourishing wholesome produce and feeling the benefits to my body and my mind over a period of time".

Amazingly, if you start to eat healthy foods on purpose, you will not only feel better, you will also lose weight. And if you are not carrying excess weight, you will find your appetite naturally dictates how much to eat to maintain your weight.

Weight – a confusing issue

What is a healthy weight for you? Please do not confuse 'ideal weight' as given in an 'average' weight/height table or BMI [Body Mass Index] with what is a healthy body weight for you personally. Differences in gender, body type and build mean that two people of the same height can have a vastly different healthy body weight.

The best way to 'know' your healthy body weight is not to know it! In other words, an arbitrary measurement on the scales is not what dictates health. Scales can be the scourge of health when people become obsessed with the pointer or electronic reading. A much better way to know and respect your body is to stand naked in front of a full-length mirror. OK, so initially you may not like what you see. However, if you take the time to learn about your relationship with food and make gradual step-by-step changes, what you see in the mirror over a period of time will be a healthier body. It can also be a more toned body as you follow the same principles for exercising which we explore in a moment.

Question yourself about your relationship with food

If you feel you have an issue with regard to eating and dieting what exactly is it? Write your answer in your letter to yourself. Try to add some thoughts on practical ways to do something differently with regard to the food you eat? If you feel it is appropriate, write a few sentences in your health letter about what you plan to change, the steps you are going to take and any ideas for support measures which will encourage you to stick with it for life.

Use the daily HELP prompt – put a copy on your fridge door

Healthy eating and drinking choices – that's what I make these days!

Enjoying my body and engaging my self-respect – it feels good!

Learning to be free of anxiety, worry and guilt over food – I'm getting there!

Positive choices for positive vital energy in my life – it's not that complicated!

A3: Your relationship with alcohol

Most of us have experienced that pleasant light-headed sensation shortly after having an alcoholic drink, particularly on an empty stomach. It feels good and our defences are lowered. We speak more freely and like the sound of our own voices. Those of us who are normally shy may feel able to come out of our shells. Those of us who are normally extrovert and supremely confident may go over the top and try to play the star role in an inappropriate manner.

Not only does a moderate amount of alcohol make us feel good, researchers have even reported that drinking a glass of red wine a day seems to be beneficial for health. Meanwhile whisky drinkers wax lyrical about anti-blood clotting properties attributed to their favourite tipple.

With pleasure comes pain

Unfortunately something as initially pleasurable and easily attainable as alcohol, has a downside. Yes, as we all know, too much alcohol is decidedly dangerous. We are not just talking about the tragedy associated with chronic alcoholism and cirrhosis of the liver. We would also like to mention the ghastly disruption of an alcoholic daze – that awful hangover, the pounding headache, the disturbed sleep, the smelly breath, the poisoned cells and the inability to concentrate at work – 'the morning after the night before'.

Be aware of your alcohol habit

Awareness is important. If you choose to drink alcohol, and many of us do, then be aware of that choice and look at it closely to determine what sort of alcohol habit you have, even if it is not a problem and you just want to keep an eye on it. But perhaps your consumption has got out of hand? In which case, this is an opportunity to re-examine your drinking habits and choose to make changes.

We say 'opportunity' because, as with all physically addictive substances, there may be a tough period of withdrawal when you need additional medical and emotional support. However strong your will is to succeed on day 1, be aware that you are susceptible to the physical and emotional temptations of alcohol for a very long time. Your doctor will advise you and there are many helpful organisations offering support both for yourself and for your relatives.

Question yourself about your relationship with alcohol

For the purposes of the 5th Enrichment Experience, let us assume that you are not out of control with alcohol but feel an appraisal of the situation could be helpful. If you have a serious alcohol addiction, please seek professional advice.

Ask yourself: "what are my issues around drinking alcohol?" Write your answer in your health letter to yourself. Try to add some thoughts on how to deal with this in a practical way.

What is your answer telling you about your current drinking habits – is there room for improvement? If you feel it is appropriate, write a sentence or two in your health letter about what you plan to change, the practical steps you are going to take and any personal support measures which will encourage you to maintain a healthy regime long-term.

Invoking willpower

It is useful to reflect that you do have the choice to control the amount of alcohol you drink. No-one else can make this choice for you. It will require both willpower and practical steps to help change an alcohol habit. *"It's not that some people have willpower and some don't. It's that some people are ready to change and others are not."* James Gordon.

A4: Are you a smoker?

If you are reading this paragraph, possibly your lungs have a relationship with tobacco fumes and tar, and your body is addicted to nicotine? Just like the previous section on alcohol, it is important to recognise the initial pleasure that smoking gives. If people didn't find smoking pleasurable, they would never become hooked on cigarettes or cigars.

Quite apart from social bans on smoking, there is a need to be realistic as to why you are considering quitting the habit. As mentioned before, you really have 'to want to be a non-smoker' to be successful. Simply acknowledging smoking is bad for you and contributes to several revolting diseases doesn't seem to work in the struggle to stop smoking.

There are many different methods to help people become non-smokers – e-cigarette vaping, acupuncture, hypnosis, nicotine substitute implants/patches, nicotine-based chewing gum, self-help support groups, online quit clubs. Ah we hear you say, "if I stop smoking, I may start eating more to compensate and end up with a weight problem". Absolutely! If you choose to eat more food than you need, you will undoubtedly put on weight but why make that choice just because you have quit smoking – there are alternatives.

Breaking that oral fixation and smoking cues

It is our belief that the relationship between smoking and eating is connected to an oral fixation which is supposed to give us some kind of uncertain satisfaction. As a society, we seem to be addicted to putting unnecessary things in our mouths – cigarettes, chewing gum, lollypops, sugary drinks, even pencils. Once you identify the nature of your own personal oral fixation then you can do something about it.

The same goes for smoking cues. As you become a non-smoker, there will be certain cues, specific to you, that tempt you to have a cigarette. For instance, being with friends who are smokers, having a cup of coffee or an alcoholic drink which you used to accompany with a cigarette. Whatever your personal cues, recognise them and develop a new mode of behaviour to pre-empt your craving.

You may choose to 'condition' yourself with a different action pattern. Every time you feel the urge to put a cigarette in your mouth, you can do one of several physical activities, depending on your immediate circumstances.

- Focus on breathing deeply for a few moments. Ideally find a quiet spot somewhere away from cars, chemicals, dust and any other obvious pollutants. Stand with feet slightly apart, your forearms held out either side, palms upwards. Alternatively sit in a comfortable chair. Slowly take a deep breath, hold to the count of five then release it slowly – all the way until your lungs feel empty. Now repeat the process; continue as long as you like. Imagine your lungs are living sponges enjoying the interaction with clean fresh air. Think about how good it feels.

- Pretend you are a professional singer and belt out a song. See how long you can hold the last note.

- Switch your immediate surroundings by crossing the floor, going into another room, going out for a run or a walk. Look around you – take in the sights and sounds.

- Change whatever it is you're doing at the time of your urge to indulge. Distract yourself with something new.

- Clean your teeth with a fresh-flavoured toothpaste – this really works! Or try a mint mouth wash.

- Chew on some low-calorie foods – carrot strips, celery, cauliflower, cucumber, peppers – which can be ready prepared in the fridge for just such an emergency.

- Suck the occasional strong mint – however be careful with chewing gum – it can leave you feeling empty and windy, plus it conditions you to feel the need to chew something all the time. This may reinforce your oral fixation – the very thing you are trying to get away from.

Other remedies include nicotine substitutes or a course of hypnosis – try a mix of whatever feels right for you.

Question yourself about your smoking habit

If you feel you have an issue with regard to smoking, exactly what is it? Write your answer in your health letter. Try to add some action points on how you can best be a non-smoker – possibly engaging some of the practical techniques above.

This is how being a non-smoker feels

You can feel high on good clean fresh air. You can feel your lungs functioning better without the presence of polluting particles. You can start to taste your food again; your skin is saved from the damaging effects of smoke; your breath is sweeter and your mouth more kissable; you even have more money in your pocket for other things like holidays; your clothes and your home smell better. Non-smokers feel released from the shackles of nicotine – it's a good feeling.

A5: Your approach to exercise

The body is a wonderful physical entity which, like a machine, needs to move around otherwise it will seize up. Today it is widely acknowledged that exercising the body is not only essential for our physical health but also for our mental health. The two are inextricably linked and the relationship between mind and body operates at all levels.

In the fast lane are the electrical impulses in your brain and spinal cord whose incredible speed gives you the ability to have almost instant reflex reactions in remote muscles – next time you touch something that is unbearably hot you'll know what we mean. Then there are molecules in our bodies, including hormones, which can act as biochemical messengers. So-called 'mental stress', for example, may affect the biochemistry of the physical body, possibly leading to 'dis-ease'. When you have a near miss in a car the adrenalin response kicks in almost instantly. It sets your heart beat racing and may make you sweat. This is the so-called 'fight or flight' reaction of primitive man – whichever he chose to do, there was some physical activity involved.

Nowadays, we still have the same adrenalin response, but often we are unable to make a physical movement to expurgate the build-up of stressful biochemical substances in our bodies – being stuck in a car is just one example. When you get angry, you may be tempted to take remedial physical action but thankfully our society does not allow you to do so. Physically allowing yourself to let off steam through exercise is the best choice every time.

The joy of movement

In the slow lane, but equally important for our mental health is the wonderful 'feel good factor' which comes from being able to enjoy moving one's body, keeping it honed and toned and healthy. And consider the world's top chess players, renowned for their exceptional mental agility. The training regime of Grand Masters recognises that physical exercise is intrinsically beneficial for intense concentration.

Hopefully you are now convinced that physical exercise is something to consider as a regular feature of your daily life. It seems to us that people and physical exercise, broadly speaking, fall into three categories – which one are you in?

Group 1: People who already enjoy regular exercise

If you fall into this group, you are probably keen to reconfirm your good feelings about physical health. That's fine, as long as you are not overdoing it to the point where exercise becomes an obsession or takes too much time away from other activities. Assuming you do regular healthy exercise, please spread the word by example and by diplomatically encouraging others to engage the exercise habit.

Group 2: People who cringe at the thought of exercise

If you are one of those people who has a perceived problem with physical exercise, please read on. We would like to introduce you to the idea that you can choose to enjoy using your body in a simple walking movement, gentle swimming, cycling on the level, maybe trying your hand at golf, or Pilates, or even something a little more aerobic, like dancing or hill-walking. Instead of thinking of exercise as the dreaded discipline or ultra-competitive lesson you were forced to do at school, choose to view it as a pleasurable way to move your body – no-one is expecting you to be an Olympian.

You could start with a simple breathing exercise coupled with some gentle movement – possibly to music. Then go for a walk in beautiful surroundings. Learn to enjoy your sense of liveliness and vitality. How about getting together with like-minded friends and sharing the experience? We guarantee you will glow in the aftermath of physical activity.

Group 3: People who like the idea but claim to be 'too busy'

Can you hear yourself saying: "it's all very well, I would love to do more exercise but I simply haven't got the time". There is a simple answer to this – make the time! How much time do you spend watching TV, reading papers or magazines or on your smart phone/the internet [other than for specific business reasons], talking unnecessarily – especially on the phone, lying in bed in the morning when you are awake?

Could you use some of this time to walk, run or swim? Could you beat the rush hour and arrange to exercise in the vicinity of your workplace before work – or after work? Could you use the stairs instead of the lift? Could you walk to and from the station? Choose to be creative with your time. If you treat it as a challenge, you will probably be able to find half hour here or there. In return, you may be adding many extra healthy months, years or even decades, to your lifespan.

Question yourself about your exercise habit

Whichever of the Groups above you identify with best, the question to ask is: "what are my issues, if any, around physical exercise?" Write your answer in your health letter.

What is your answer telling you about your current exercise habit or lack of it – is there room for improvement? Can you find ways to optimise the amount of daily/weekly exercise you do, or want to do in future. If you feel it is appropriate, write a few words about the practical steps you can take to increase the amount of exercise you take. This may include finding opportunities for exercising in company or other support measures which will encourage you to stick with it.

Start today

Your body is meant to move [a lot], so here is a paradoxical quote from J. R. R. Tolkien to fire you up to enjoy a physical celebration of your body: *"It is the job that is never started that takes the longest to finish."* Make sure you 'start' today!

A6: Your sleep pattern

The quality and quantity of sleep is intrinsically linked to your overall health. Memory, creativity and mood are all serviced by a good night's sleep. The question of sleep is however totally individual so there are no hard and fast rules. Some people appear to thrive on around five hours a night, while most of us need an average of seven to eight hours. Some people nod off during the day and then complain they have difficulty sleeping through the night; others call it 'a power nap' and claim it invigorates them for the rest of the day.

Keep to a regular routine

The latest research from the US on sleep emphasises the importance of a regular sleep routine. Keeping to the same bedtime and waking time [and nap time if appropriate] seems to be extremely beneficial because the body functions best in a state of homeostasis. As anyone who has experienced jet lag will know, being out of kilter with your personal body clock can leave you feeling out of sorts, even quite unwell. It has also been documented that variable shift workers generally have a shorter life expectancy than an equivalent age/social status control group.

Sleep upsets

People who indulge in large meals, drink strong coffee, watch violent TV programmes or engage in intense physical activity late at night, may experience sleep disturbance. Then there are those who unnaturally force themselves to stay awake into the wee small hours for matters of social convenience or digital addiction with the result that their sleep patterns become erratic.

Alcohol is an enigmatic factor when it comes to sleep. Acting as a depressant on the nervous system, alcohol can make you feel sleepy. Whereas you may experience no trouble in falling asleep, you may well toss and turn later in the night as your liver struggles to deal with the toxins.

Worry is another big sleep assassinator. Lying in bed at night is often a time for re-assessing the day's events or even your life events. With the 'wrong' kind of thinking, you may start to worry over things you cannot possibly do anything about while you are supposed to be sleeping. Stress at work, overwork, financial worries, family tensions, personal problems can all surface and disrupt your sleep.

Question yourself about your sleep patterns

If you are not getting enough rest then play detective on your particular sleep patterns and ask yourself what you believe is behind them? How does your current lifestyle impact your sleep? For instance: interruptive noise [partner snoring, noisy neighbours, you live near an airport or busy road], sharing a bed/duvet with a restless sleeper, too much light in the bedroom, late supper, alcohol overindulgence, worry, using light-intensive screens in bed? Write your answers in your health letter and add some thoughts about how best to deal with any sleep issues in a practical way.

Find your best sleep enhancers

Once you have identified the aspects of your lifestyle which impact your ability to sleep soundly, you can make some changes and introduce natural sleep enhancing measures as opposed to pharmaceutical sleeping pills. Listen to your body and common sense will guide you. If you are sleepless in the middle of the night, it is sometimes better to read for a while [not on a screen], rather than force yourself to try and fall asleep. What is important is that you are physically as well as mentally rested. *"Sleep is that golden chain that ties health and our bodies together."* Thomas Dekker.

A7: Cleansing, massaging and generally caring for your body

Looking after your body is generally talked about in terms of eating and exercise. However, setting aside reasonable time to cleanse, care and massage your body is also an integral part of healthy living. It is often done absent-mindedly or as a chore. We suggest you take time to do it 'on purpose'.

The range of pleasant smelling perfumes and deodorants, bath/shower products and massage oils is gargantuan, so you can experiment with different fragrances. Try to source natural ones rather than artificial chemical substitutes.

Think about the ambience of the room you are in for your cleansing. How about a change of décor? Could the lighting be more relaxing? Have you ever tried taking a bath by candlelight? How about introducing some water music? Let that warm shower spray caress your head, your shoulders, your lower back and your genitals.

Know your own body like the back of your hand

You can choose to use your cleansing time to get to know your body better, particularly if you are embarking on a healthy eating and exercise way of life – you can enjoy seeing the improvements as you go along.

You can also make a thorough monthly check for any irregularities. If you are female, check your breasts and if you are male, check your testes. If you notice anything unusual consult your doctor right away. The same goes for moles and skin blemishes – if you notice moles that are irregular, bleed, change colour, grow or itch, seek medical advice as soon as possible.

Likewise, warts in the genital region should be treated by a qualified medical practitioner who will also recommend a cervical smear test for women. This is a precautionary measure to check for abnormal cells at the neck of the womb that sometimes occur in conjunction with the human genital wart virus. This particular virus is now common in the sexually active population and is therefore not a stigma. It is quite possible for the virus to be present without any sign of actual warts. A simple test can determine this.

Other genital or urinary symptoms, including unpleasant discharges, should be reported to your doctor or the appropriate clinic where your confidentiality is respected. It goes without saying that you should never have unprotected sex with anyone other than a safe regular partner. Dealing with these matters is simply part of being a responsible person who takes care of their body – after all it's the only one you've got. There are lots of pleasant things you can do with it too! One of them is to develop your sense of touch.

A touching experience

Hugging and touching – they are free and easy to do. For some of us, social convention or parental influence may have suppressed our natural proclivity for physical contact so we are shy and awkward about being tactile.

In fact, keeping a stiff upper lip, being socially reserved and hiding emotions were all considered appropriate ways to conduct oneself until the liberating 1960s. Thankfully most of us are now awake to the benefits of touch and there is even empirical evidence as to its benefits. Medical research has come up with the finding that stroking a pet increases your chances of recovery after a heart attack. The relaxing influence of the tactile sense is assumed to play a part.

If your partner, family member or a friend is available, you can take it in turns to deliver a relaxing massage. [NB We are not referring here to massage of a sexual nature or for serious physiotherapeutic reasons.] There are many books on the subject of massage, some of which will come under the heading of aromatherapy. You can heighten your massage experience by using essential oils or body lotion.

It is important to feel comfortable either giving or receiving the massage. This means being both psychologically happy about it and physically comfortable in terms of your standing, kneeling or bending position, or your lying position, and the room temperature should be ambient for relaxation. Even if the room temperature is pleasant, cold hands or cold body lotion onto a warm back can invoke immediate tenseness – exactly the opposite effect to that intended.

Question yourself about body care and tactile habits

If you have any issues with regard to caring for your body, what exactly are they? Can you identify practical ways to improve your body maintenance? If you want, write a few words in your health letter about what you plan to change.

Feel clean and vibrant

The pay-off for keeping in touch with your body is a vibrancy that radiates to others. In the same way as we sometimes stop and smell the flowers, people are drawn to individuals who espouse clean healthy living – let it be you.

A8: Your attitude to stress and how it impacts your health

As we have already discussed in Chapter 7 [Part 1], your mental and physical health are inextricably linked, including the ways in which you experience 'stress' and handle stressful situations. It is vital to recognise what 'pushes your buttons' when you feel stressed – some people refer to this as 'the red mist'. Developing an appropriate response in stressful situations is critical for your long-term well-being. A healthy response goes hand in glove with good attitude and acceptance of 'what is', however tense you may feel.

Stress comes to our minds and bodies through various channels – physical injury, psychological pressure, allergic reaction, infectious illness, hormonal dysfunction, toxic exposure, poor quality food and drink, email overload, sleep deprivation – there's even a term doing the rounds called 'hurry sickness' – are any of these familiar to you?

De-stress not distress – your choice!

Too much of the so-called stress hormone cortisol in our bodies – built up over a period of time – can result in all kinds of 'distress', aches and pains, even serious illness. This distress can include tension headaches, panic attacks, irritable bowel syndrome, or even pretending we are doing well while keeping secrets, possibly telling lies to save face.

And being stressed affects our behaviour – we may comfort eat or drink too much or take recreational drugs or become sexually reckless or isolate ourselves from social encounters – which in turn may lead to even more stress. Yet the bottom line is that, for whatever reason, we have chosen these behaviours, so by implication we are free to choose an alternative strategy for keeping tension at bay. Note: we also cover aspects of relaxation and meditation in the 7th and 8th Enrichment Experiences, which gives you further scope for progress using stress-reducing techniques.

Plenty of information – but where to start?

Books and articles on stress are incredibly popular today and you may well have been motivated by them. Perhaps you have attended a stress management seminar with the aim of enhancing your performance, particularly at work. However good your intent, stress management strategies in isolation cannot always blend in with your 'real world' experiences. Demanding children, physical illness, an unsympathetic boss, a sense of having no control, lack of time to get everything done [even after you've reorganised your schedule in line with the advice of a course, book or article] – all contrive to sabotage resolutions.

The best way to switch off and relax is an entirely personal matter. Relaxation doesn't necessarily mean doing nothing, in fact your relaxation could be a fairly intense hobby – anything that takes you away from the stresses and strains of your normal routine. A sports hobby, for instance, would be our idea of relaxation but it might not be yours – everyone to their own. Perhaps you would like to test the maxim 'a change is as good as a rest' and find daily mini-changes that help you to keep tension at bay?

Question yourself about the stress in your life

If you feel you have an issue with stress, exactly what is it? You will need to be open with yourself about your lifestyle and your personality. Write about your stress situation in your health letter. Try to add some thoughts on how to deal with this in a practical way.

Stress free living – oh what joy!

Use your initiative and insight to reach the stage where you appreciate relaxation or other anti-stress activities of your choice as being 'on purpose', and look forward to relieving tension in a proactive way on a daily basis. It is in our own best interests to find a happy medium – a balanced way of living which is exciting and relaxing, dutiful and rewarding.

Back to your all-embracing Health Letter

As you write your heath letter incorporating as many, or as few, of the health issues raised in the 5th Enrichment Experience, you may find yourself prompted to radically re-think your current lifestyle. Alternatively, you may just want to bring a few healthier options into your daily regime. Whatever your reasoning, now is as good a time as any to get started. So write your intent in a constructive way avoiding negativity – you can add to it anytime.

Headline your final paragraph: "Glad to be alive." Now choose three things, related to the 5th Enrichment, that 'make your heart sing'. They could be an appreciation of your physical and mental health and any plans for major changes to reinvigorate your life. An easy way to do this is to finish the sentence: "I'm glad that ......"

Put your completed letter in an envelope [preferably of your favourite colour] and place it in the centre of your home. The significance of this will become apparent in ACTION B.

ACTION B: Create an inspiring environment

To what extent is your physical and mental well-being affected by your surroundings? Is there any difference to your health between being in a dingy cluttered damp smelly house or a clean, tidy, cosy well-lit one? When you go out for a walk, would you rather be on a country path or a traffic snarled urban road?

The 5th Enrichment emphasises the importance of choosing to live and work in supportive environments that enhance your opportunities for good health and quality of life. In addition, we specifically urge you to think about what exists at the heart of everything – the centre of our minds, bodies, and homes. According to ancient wisdom, this is where the potential for harmony, unity and balance resides. Known as the Tai Chi, the centre is represented by the union of yin and yang energies, said to comprise the entire universe.

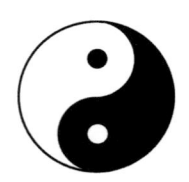

The circular yin-yang symbol with its intertwined black and white elements, plus a tiny circle of yin in the yang and a tiny circle of yang in the yin, illustrates how harmony is achieved through the interdependence of complementary opposites.

In so-called 'western societies', we are raised to view 'opposites' as being totally dissimilar from each other. By contrast, eastern philosophy advises us that opposites are best viewed as being complementary. They are part of the same whole – we cannot know hot without knowing cold, up or down, hard or soft, hate or love, motion or stillness, war or peace, stress or relaxation. We are urged to find the harmonious middle way for our human endeavours.

So let's look to the centre of our homes for inspiration. Metaphorically this is where we 'earth ourselves' – the ground on which we lay the foundations for a meaningful life. Locate the centre of your home and think about the significance of this area for you. Is it an open space or a small closet, a storeroom or a place of relaxation, the kitchen at the hub of family life or a quiet reflective space?

Clearing central clutter supports your health intentions

First remove any clutter or ugly items, and re-organise any storage that has got out of hand. For instance, if the centre of your home happens to be the under stairs cupboard, please take everything out and re-arrange it practically and beautifully. Wherever your centre is located, it can be absolutely gorgeous, clutter free and inviting.

Focus Features – placing on purpose – physical reminders

Apart from a general tidy up, the centre of your home is a good place to feel grounded. This can be achieved by displaying 'earth objects' and decoratively using 'earthy colours and textures'. For this purpose, earth is said to be represented by ceramics, gems, stones, rocks, pebbles, soil, sand, gravel, yellow or brown objects and décor, and paintings or photographs that contain these elements.

In addition, earth is supported by the fire element, so a splash of red, a bright light or a fireplace are all useful symbolically.

However these are mere suggestions. Most importantly, because the centre of your home represents complete union, it can be decorated any which way 'feels good to you personally'. You might also like to paint a black/white yin-yang symbol on a smooth pebble or create a yin-yang picture to grace your wall. It can act as a reminder that good health emanates from living in a balanced way – mind, body and spirit in harmony with the environment.

ACTION C: Three ways to wellness diagram

This health exercise is something of an exception to the non-prescriptive approach that we adhere to in the Habitat Affect. For this reason, it is more likely to appeal to those of you who thrive when given specific directions!

Get into a comfortable position that allows you to draw and write easily.

Have a blank piece of paper or card and some coloured pens at the ready.

Start by reading the following 3 directives and their rationale:

[1] Show respect for your body

Feed your body with wholesome nourishing foods – choose not to put unhealthy junk food into yourself. Your amazing body deserves only the best. The same goes for liquids and other substances. Every single day, make sure you use your body properly. This means undertaking physical exercise, even if you can only manage walking. Human bodies are not meant to be static. If we continually abuse them by remaining in fixed positions for long periods of time, not only will they start to hurt but also our mental well-being will be compromised. If you live a sedentary existence, without a reasonable amount of physical activity – that is your choice. But do not be surprised if your life reflects your inactivity in other ways. There are many different types of exercise – you need to find a regime that suits your individual lifestyle – a physical way of relating to your body that becomes second nature to you.

[2] Show respect for your mind

Feed your mind with the information that you need to develop calm wisdom and useful know-how. Employ personal discipline when it comes to your reading material and choice of TV viewing or internet browsing. Avoid idle chatter. Indulge a healthy sense of humour. Sit in silence at least once a day to energise your spirit. Make learning a life-long experience. You can learn from young and old alike. Be selective. Without preaching, pass on your know-how and wisdom by example. And remember to cultivate patience.

[3] Rejoice in the fact that you are alive

First thing in the morning when you awake, take a deep breath, a liberating body stretch and just feel the life force energy surging through you. Start the day with an inspiring thought and a smile. When you can see the silver linings of your personal rain clouds, indulge this vision. Pass on your wisdom to others by example and share your passion for the welfare of the planet. Always remember to celebrate your good fortune as it manifests by saying 'thank you' for the gift of life when something marvellous comes along.

Sign-up

Now you can 'sign up' to these three aspirations by making a personal wellness diagram.

Draw a circle in the middle of a sheet of paper or card and inside write the words 'my amazing health-giving life' or choose whatever words feel right for you.

Draw three wide 'roads' all leading to the circle and label them: I respect my body; I respect my mind; I'm glad to be alive. Embellish and decorate your diagram with words and images of your choice.

Display your diagram in a suitable place as an aide memoir. Look at your diagram often, keep on track, feel good about yourself and smile!

ACTION D: Make a difference – change something

This is your chance to commit to change something for the better. Perhaps write down what you intend to do and give yourself an achievable time schedule. Decide on a Focus Feature for your home that will help to motivate you.

Health is a lifelong journey, so any changes you choose to make are likely to be ongoing and evolutionary. Whatever you decide to do, make sure it is in tune with the essence of the 5th Enrichment – that is to participate fully in your physical and mental health for your own personal benefit and, by example, to inspire everyone with whom you connect to join the good health journey.

THE 6th ENRICHMENT EXPERIENCE

Friendship; guides; helpful people; offering help to others; care for the environment; leisure and social time; travel and adventures; appreciation. *"Real happiness in life starts when you begin to cherish others."* Lama Zopa Rinpoche.

It is remarkable just how many words beginning with 'C' are ideal for describing the attributes of great friendships and generally enhancing our interactions with others. Here are a few 'C' words in random order – maybe you can add more.

Communication – two-way communication, with attentive listening, is at the very heart of robust loyal friendships.

Contribution – our offer of help at both personal – friends and family – and community level for the benefit of others.

Care – for the environment, acknowledging the essential role of creatures and plants with whom we share the earth.

Courage – having the courage of one's convictions to speak out for what is right in society and to act responsibly.

Consideration – to ensure our actions do not knowingly harm others, always allowing for unintended consequences.

Compassion – showing empathy and kindness, even when we have been hurt, knowing there is usually a silver lining.

Concern – for those we love when they are ill or in difficulty which can often best be shown in practical ways.

Courtesy – to be polite and well-mannered as a mark of respect; having a courteous attitude works for both parties.

Compliments – giving them is free and people appreciate being appreciated. Compliment-givers feel good too!

The 6th Enrichment Experience is about your life based around friendship – for people and the planet – and the time you spend on leisure and social activities, including travel and adventures. Our intellectual and emotional development is enriched by involvement with others from childhood right through to our vintage years. Every time we offer support and encouragement to someone else, we also contribute to our own well-being. Here we look at aspects of this important, yet sometimes overlooked, part of life.

The value of friendships

As Rumi so delightfully said: *"You may be happy enough going along, but with others you'll get farther and faster."*

True friendship always requires two-way traffic – giving and receiving, listening and talking, comforting and being comforted, having fun and laughing together. It also requires time and effort. Taking people for granted is not the way to sustain friendship. Indeed, there are times when we need to make special effort and go the extra mile. But this is well worth it, for being in harmony with other people is both pleasurable and a key constituent of good mental health. If you are interested in developing your listening skills [an important aspect of friendship], please visit Appendix I.

Occasionally we need to assess friendships and possibly cull those which no longer serve us or the other person. Deciding we have outgrown a friendship is a highly personal matter. Our interests and circumstances are constantly evolving. While 'shared history' is brilliant for those cradle-to-grave type friendships, there are others we enter along the way and then fail to exit at the appropriate moment.

Making new friends and acquaintances

There are occasions when we feel the need to cultivate new friends. This is particularly an issue for people whose job mobility takes them far away from their friends and original communities. Making new friends requires a certain degree of confidence and is best achieved through shared interests.

The internet now provides those of us who find ourselves in remote locations with the possibility of instant access to close friends when we are geographically separated. Sadly there can also be a downside to internet friendships when people spend valuable leisure time with casual 'virtual friends in virtual worlds' to the exclusion of personal human contact. This may lead to an unhealthy isolating existence.

Differentiating between friends and mere acquaintances is also important. It is only possible to have a few close friends because such friendships require service time. Some people claim to have many friends but really they are talking about acquaintances. It's a helpful distinction, especially when we are feeling lonely and in need of true friends – one will do!

Whether friend, work colleague or passing acquaintance, we can always give the person a dose of our appreciation. In the wise words of Voltaire *"Appreciation is a wonderful thing. It makes what is excellent in others belong to us as well."*

Are you a friend of the earth?

Broadening the friendship arena to social and environmental responsibility – to be a friend of all humankind and creature-kind – we need to be a friend of the earth. Caring for the environment, in however small a way, is part of our legacy for the next generation – our children and grandchildren.

Our use of energy, our methods of transport, our food production, the excessive use of pesticides and fertilizers, the pollution of our rivers with antibiotic residues and household-cleaning chemicals, the financial products we invest in, the manufacture of our clothes, the trading arrangements we sanction, our attitudes to packaging and the discarding of waste – all these and more are the responsibility of governments and of individuals like us.

However we must avoid engaging in a massive guilt trip that could paralyse us into doing nothing. When there is so much to be done, it can seem like an insurmountable dilemma. Realistically, we are all part of the problem, which means we are also capable of being part of the solution.

Living in an eco-conscious way requires quite a bit of effort and we cannot expect to go from zero to perfect overnight. First we need to be aware of the issues, to think about where we stand on them and then choose to be actively eco-friendly in those areas we feel are worthwhile – the ones we are capable of sustaining. In the words of Mahatma Gandhi *"Live simply so that others might simply live."*

Travel broadens the mind

Visiting and exploring countries other than our own, gives us an entirely different perspective on life. Often this can make us more appreciative of what we have back home. It is also beneficial for us as human beings to have a break from routine – the mundane ordinariness of our everyday existence – we need adventures. Going away on holiday can be like an elixir to our energy levels, we return home refreshed and reinvigorated.

Currently there is a heated debate going on about air travel and our carbon footprint with regard to global warming. Financial constraints aside, it is up to each of us to decide how much air travel we allow ourselves, and whether or not we take active steps to make reparations. For example, we can choose to make charitable contributions towards tree-planting, agricultural schemes, water purification plants or educational projects, in the countries we visit. We could try an alternative method of transport – take a train for instance.

Some of us prefer to travel alone and meet people along the way. For others, sharing the sights, sounds, tastes and smells of foreign lands with a partner or friend is a wonderful experience. Travel and adventure go hand in hand. But for those who are averse to travel, it is also possible to take an adventure in the mind by reading a good book, watching a travelogue or movie, or by indulging in creative writing.

Your leisure and social life

This is the area of your life that is easy to neglect, especially when things become hectic at work or when you become subservient to the time constraints of another person.

By 'work' we mean everything connected with your work, such as staying late at the office, bringing work home, using your smart phone to check messages out of working hours, being stuck in a traffic jam on the way to and from work, feeling trapped at home with a couple of demanding children and piles of housework to get through. It's at times like these you really crave some 'spare time', some proper leisure time. "Spare time – I haven't got time for any!" – does this sound like you?

Ironically, when faced with this very same 'spare time', some of us have a tendency to sabotage our own relaxation and play the working martyr – yes human beings are a strange lot. How many people do you know who make hard work of holidays? Are you one of them? Or are you jeopardising your recreational activities by choosing to allow one insular relationship to monopolise your time, when you could be spending some of it with supportive friends?

Insomuch as your leisure and social time includes your health and relationships, it is a major part of your life. And it seems to be the case that people with robust social ties are motivated to take good care of themselves. Social interactions, at work or play, can help to nurture self-esteem and bolster a beneficial feeling that one's life is significant.

Purposefully spending time alone – solitude as opposed to loneliness – is also beneficial, and your true friends will understand this. Today we often refer to the desire for solitude as 'needing some space', which you can read about in the 8th Enrichment Experience.

Couch potato or active leisure lover

Your experience of life is founded to a great extent on how you choose to spend your time. If you consciously focus on making preparations for quality leisure time, this can have a massive influence on your enjoyment of life and sociability.

Person A: You're exhausted after a busy day at work. You get home at about 19.00 hours, having been caught up in rush hour traffic. You pour yourself a drink, and sit down in front of the TV. You may even eat your evening meal in front of a screen. The conversation between you and your partner, or you and your children, is limited to mundane pleasantries "Did you have a good day?" etc.

Person B: You're exhausted after a busy day at work. You get home at about 19.00 hours, having been caught up in rush hour traffic. You go upstairs and wash off the daily grime, change your clothes and play with the children or go to the gym or help to prepare a meal with your partner or go out to night school etc.

These two very simplistic illustrations serve to show that our circumstances do not ultimately dictate what happens because we all have some freedom of choice. Person A actually chose to be a couch potato, although he or she was not aware of it at the time. Person B chose to freshen up and make a few physical changes before embarking on the new evening ahead. Note the use of simple 'physical' actions such as washing and changing clothes which help to refresh the mind into a rewarding leisure mode.

The rationale for art and music and so much more

The importance of choosing to spend leisure time in the company of friends and family, or alone, or experiencing the wonders of the world, should not be underestimated. For reasons that are not completely understood, time spent on leisure activities can significantly contribute to our welfare.

The question "What use is art?" illustrates the inherent desire of people to dress up their humdrum existence to make life more pleasurable. Art, in itself, is of no obvious survival use unless you are a commercial art dealer using it to make a living. Yet 'a thing of beauty is a joy to behold'.

One of the things that early primitive people accomplished was art – as the remarkable cave drawings around the world show us. Why did they bother? The same goes for music. Why do you bother to do anything other than sleep, eat, drink, work and have sex? These basic functions would, after all, see you through. Clearly most of us feel they are not enough to keep our minds healthy and nourished. We

THE HABITAT AFFECT

seem to need involvement with art and music and books and films as our entertainment panacea for a beautiful life.

Schedule your engagements – on purpose

If you are struggling to meet friendship, leisure and social commitments that you know can make your life more pleasant, we recommend you keep a daily written diary or e-organiser and purposely schedule in all your social and hobby activities. Include a daily walk or other exercise, against a particular time slot.

If you use a paper diary, a good tip is to use coloured pens to denote your activities. For example, work appointments can be recorded in red, daily exercise [even if it is a reminder to go for a walk] can be in green. Social and relationship activities can be in blue, use black for miscellaneous appointments eg. doctor, dentist. And if you are so minded, use a purple pen for making an appointment with yourself – your alone time!

Too busy to have a happy balanced life?

Today many people choose to live in a very 'busy' way – the core ingredient of their lives being work, extra overtime work, housework, computer and smartphone interface. This is life without the social and leisure dressing.

Bringing the attributes of the 6th Enrichment into your life will help to add the dressing, the spice, the zest that makes us interesting and interested, helpful and appreciative human beings. *"Those who bring sunshine into the lives of others, cannot keep it from themselves."* J M Barrie.

The 6th Enrichment Experience Action Area

The following suggestions may help you discover what, if anything, you could change in your current routine to enhance your enjoyment of social and leisure activities, and for opportunities to safeguard the health of the planet. Choose actions that resonate with you, disregard the rest.

ACTION A: Questions & answers – your motivating letter

Write yourself a personal letter [Dear Me . . . and the date] in which you answer one or more of the following questions:

Thinking about your opportunities for time to spend with friends, leisure activities, travel and adventure, do you feel you are making the most of them?

What are your most enjoyable leisure activities and are you doing them enough?

Do you consider the welfare of the eco-system in your neighbourhood and the planet in general?

Have your answers highlighted areas where you could benefit from spending more time with friends, have a change of scenery or introduce some eco-friendly behaviour? It may be that any changes you decide to make involve clawing back some time from another area of your life or even from another leisure activity currently taking up a disproportionate amount of your time.

Try to be practical within your available time frame. With the best will in the world, without a hands-on plan you will probably revert to former ways. Maybe write a few words about what you would like to do over the next few months.

Headline your final paragraph with the words "Glad to be alive." Choose three things, related in some way to the 6th Enrichment, that 'make your heart sing'. For instance, the pleasure of confiding in a loyal friend, of being able to travel to interesting places, or having the opportunity to get involved with an environmental project. An easy way to do this is to finish the sentence: "I'm glad that ...."

Put your completed letter in an envelope [preferably white] and place it in the north west of an appropriate room in your home. The significance of this is discussed in ACTION B.

ACTION B: Create an inspiring environment

The north west of your property is the area that symbolically represents the support of guides and helpful friends, being a loyal friend to others, and good energy for travel. Solidarity and robustness typify the approach to clearing and placing Focus Features in honour of the 6th Enrichment which is associated with the metal element. This means avoiding higgledy-piggledy arrangements in favour of strong clear-cut features, furniture, colour and display.

Clearing away any hindering clutter

Is anything cluttering up your friendship, leisure and travel area? Have a look around the north west of your home or the north west of your living room and you will know intuitively if you need to have a blitz. Ideally remove every single item from the area and then replace only those items that are really necessary. Part of your clearance could be to create a clean-look by painting the walls white and observe how different a blank canvas feels.

Focus Features – placing on purpose – physical reminders

With your clean-look north west ready to receive, here are some ideas for this area or whichever part of your home you personally choose to pay tribute to friends and adventures, social activities and the earth. These suggestions are not meant to be prescriptive, just do what feels good for you, one or two things at a time.

- Display a photograph or cluster of photographs of your friends, ideally with you in the picture as well – white, silver or gold frames are best.

- Display an object given to you by a close friend, but only if you like it.

- A metal wind chime playing here is said to bring helpful people into your life.

- Place a totem animal or angel symbol to remind you of the unseen support of your sixth sense guides.

- If there is room, a table on which to do hobbies or to play cards or games with friends, could be situated here.

- Display a world map and/or arrange your travel books beautifully. Plan you next holiday with friends or family, or use a reputable solo travel company if you are single, so you have the benefit of like-minded companions.

- If you have mementos of a holiday including scenic photos, this is an ideal area to exhibit them.

- White, silver and gold décor and solid metallic objects are considered to be auspicious in this area.

- Provide illumination with a metal-based lamp or candle stick to enliven the north west.

- If you are looking for improvements in your social life, write your intentions on a piece of white paper using a silver or gold pen, date it and seal into a white envelope. Place the envelope on a metal plate or bowl. [This also applies to the personal letter you may have written in Action A]. Open the envelope in three weeks and note what has changed in your life.

ACTION C: 'Are you enjoying yourself?'

Would you like to change the amount of time you choose to spend on various social and leisure activities? Here is one way to find out by using our Enjoyment Rating System.

Everyone reading this is going to have a unique set of leisure and social activities, some of which may also be personal relationship and health issues. This exercise aims to establish how you currently choose to spend your leisure time with an enjoyment rating alongside. This will help you determine any areas where something different is called for.

Start by identifying your current leisure and social activities by selecting the activities you currently participate in from the list below. Give yourself an Enjoyment Rating on a scale of 1 to 5: where: 1 = 'I really enjoy this activity'; 2 = 'I feel this activity is fairly enjoyable'; 3 = 'I can take it or leave it'; 4 = 'I find time spent this way is not very enjoyable'; 5 = 'I really dislike spending time this way'. NB: it may be helpful to include a brief description of what you actually do during your stated leisure activities.

Activity Description

Spending time with immediate family and close relatives
Spending time together with friends – going out or staying in
Spending time alone out of choice
Watching TV/listening to specific radio programmes
Internet/smart phone – social networking/skype/gaming/other
Theatre/cinema/art/music/concerts/festivals etc
Exercise/walking/sports – watching/participating
Creative projects – crafts, cooking, sewing, writing etc
Pets – dogs, cats, horse riding etc
DIY and building projects
Non-essential shopping

Learning a foreign language for fun
Environmental projects
Religious/spiritual observance
Non-essential pampering/massage/spa treatments
Holidays at home/abroad
Reading
Gardening
Gambling
Playing cards or board games
Other ………………………………………..

Has participating in this Enjoyment Rating exercise given you a clearer view of how you currently choose to spend your leisure and social time? What does your Enjoyment Rating list look like? Have you given any of your current activities a 3, 4 or 5 rating? If so, would you like to re-view the time you spend on them or your attitude towards them? Are you giving enough time to activities you rated as 1 or 2? Are there any activities you are not currently engaging in, but would like to in future?

Doing something entirely new is a fantastic way to revitalise yourself and meet other pioneering spirits. There are, of course, only 24 hours in a day/night, so you need to find the 'right balance' for all the things you intend to do. To get things in perspective you could ask "Am I choosing to spend my leisure and social time in the best way for my welfare?"

ACTION D: Make a difference – change something

When you acknowledge the 6th Enrichment principles of healthy friendships, social activity, travel, care and respect for the earth, you are giving yourself the power to make reasoned choices, even if you have a restricted time-frame.

As inevitably your circumstances change, so you can re-think your options and activities. Only you know what is possible and what is really right for you. So make your commitment to do something differently for today, tomorrow and next week – write down your intention. Be prepared to make other longer-term changes as and when you feel they are needed. And try to remind yourself daily that *'life is a wonderful gift to be treasured and shared'*.

THE 7th ENRICHMENT EXPERIENCE

Creativity and bringing projects to completion; overcoming procrastination; harvesting; celebration; relaxation; luck of children; family time; fun; surprises. *"From little acorns, mighty oak trees grow."* Proverb.

The 7th Enrichment Experience is quite diverse in scope but basically the overall theme honours our creative nature in all its many guises. We are encouraged to put in the effort required to nurture our creative projects throughout their growth – whether at work or at home – and to harvest them when they come to fruition. Then we can take time to relax and celebrate our achievements, before embarking on the next project and so forth.

We can witness the seeds of our own human creativity by watching children absorbed in creative play. We too, as adults, can still be creative and playful. We can choose to retain or rediscover our childhood passion for inventiveness and making things, or we can allow our initiative to be stifled in the mediocre world of dead end occupation, crass TV, smartphone overuse, unnecessary shopping or mindless gossip. It is, after all, our choice.

The opening premise of the 7th Enrichment confirms there is a great sense of happiness inherent to employing our immense capacity for creativity and, specifically, by having a creative project always on the go. Being creative invigorates us and gives us a sense of achievement. Thinking, writing, drawing, painting, composing, singing, acting, theorising, debating, cooking, sewing, knitting, carving, sculpting, reproducing, decorating, making or doing something 'new to you' or, in rare instances, something new to the world – there is a wealth of choice for being creative.

Do you know your creative self?

We all have the ingredients for creativity in us and the potential to exercise our creative muscles. However some people find it easier than others to engage in creative pursuits and there are any number of reasons why our creativity sometimes gets side-lined.

We may have been conditioned by our background and education to feel most comfortable when we are following in the herd, doing the same as everyone else. Or we have got a good excuse for why we do not innovate as much as we could – too little time, it takes too much effort, fear of not being 'good enough', fear of embarrassment, fear of failure, fear of being unoriginal, no-one to do it with etc. These blocks to our innate creativity are denying us a raft of great experiences and achievements that enhance our well-being.

A brief word about effort

The media is full of stories about creative types who have seemingly come from nowhere – overnight 'effortless' sensations – to hit the headlines as artists, singers, actors, musicians, dancers etc. The truth is that most of these people have been working hard behind the scenes and have often had to overcome rejection on many occasions – that is the bit we do not see. They have continued to believe in themselves and their creativity despite numerous set-backs.

On the other hand, there are hundreds of very talented people who either expect the world to come to them or procrastinate and never get off the bottom rung of the ladder. What we learn from this is that bringing creative projects to completion requires dedicated sustained effort, sometimes over several years.

For those of you looking for smaller scale more immediate results, there are any number of worthwhile creative projects always available. For instance, you can paint a picture at night school or write an article for the local newspaper, make a cushion cover or take part in the local amateur dramatic performance – put in the appropriate effort and you will experience the creative feel-good factor first hand.

Procrastination versus a sense of achievement

"Attention is the rarest and purest form of generosity" Simon Weil. This being so, are you paying attention to the needs of your creative self? Are you being generous to yourself with regard to managing your time productively so that you complete whatever it is you set your mind to?

If you are genuinely interested in releasing more of your creativity, then you may like to start by confronting the tendency to procrastinate. As many of us have experienced, procrastination surfaces in all sorts of guises and is the enemy of creativity. Let us assume for a moment that you are a bit of a procrastinator who wants to change! Great news: the feel-good factor of accomplishment – a glowing sense of achievement – is available to everyone whether they are experimenting with a recipe, throwing a pot, writing a bestseller or winning an Oscar.

The common denominator is that everyone who involves themselves with their creative side is overcoming their fear of failure and actually doing something. Writers write, painters paint, weavers weave and procrastinators – you guessed it – they talk about writing, painting, weaving or whatever and then, talk some more. As Jung said *"you are what you do, not what you say you'll do"*.

Of course it is very easy to procrastinate. So what's a good way to get into action mode? It is a bit like baking bread, you have to break it up into tasks, then each task becomes a workable step. If you want to learn about tasking in more detail, see if you can match the development and progression of a creative idea with the description of bread-making in Appendix J, which includes a list of task-based ingredients for harnessing creativity through to completion.

Luck of children

Parenthood is possibly the ultimate expression of creativity – bringing into existence the miracle of a new human being. In the 7th Enrichment Experience we call this 'luck of children'. Even if you do not have children of your own, you can still experience 'luck of children' by enjoying the company of those children you do come into contact with – as nieces, nephews, cousins and little friends.

We are asking you to think about how children enrich your life, even if it is sometimes in the way their presence challenges you to develop a keener sense of tolerance and patience? We are not denying that children can be a source of annoyance at certain times, but our irritation can tell us quite a bit about ourselves.

On a positive note, interacting with children can be extremely liberating as we re-engage our playful nature and let go of our inhibitions – when was the last time you were really silly in a fun way?

When it comes to love – such is the depth of the love of a parent for their child that it is impossible to describe in words. For those of us lucky enough to know and feel this love, we can give thanks and radiate loving energy in our interactions with adults and children alike.

The family unit

From the procreation of children also comes the creation of a new unit – the family. We all have experience of a family unit of one kind or another. This is something we may take for granted but it is paramount to our well-being that we live, for the most part, in harmony with other family members.

Those of us who have grown up in supportive entertaining fun environments will know the warm glowing feeling of being part of a happy family. Ideally, everyone in the family understands that when things do get out of balance, there is an unwritten agreement to find an amicable solution and return to harmony. *"Never let the sun go down on your anger"* is a maxim that works for families if they are to thrive and support the well-being of each individual member.

Poor quality family relationships and family feuds, on the other hand, are notoriously stressful – in particular the breakdown of family life during separation and divorce. This subject is not specifically covered herein, however throughout this book, you can find helpful suggestions about living your life as best as you can, even during such difficult periods. If you are going through a truly testing time, you may find that seeking professional mediation will help you and other family members to agree on arrangements that produce a feasible balance for all concerned.

Celebrate something

Another aspect of the 7th Enrichment Experience is celebration. Society gives us special days on which to celebrate – national holidays and festivals, birthdays and anniversaries are all part of the annual calendar of events. Then there are life's landmark celebrations from academic, sporting or musical achievements to competence in our field of work and chosen hobbies.

We champion the idea that everyday gives us the chance to celebrate something – even if it is just the fact that we woke up this morning and can feel the life force flowing through us with the potential to create something in this new day.

As everyone's idea of celebration is different, we leave the mechanics of how you choose to celebrate entirely up to you. Celebration could mean anything from an extreme activity holiday, having friends over for supper or a long soak in a perfumed bath by candlelight.

The point is that celebration is done on purpose – we acknowledge the occasion or achievement to be honoured and then devise a suitable way to express our celebration.

Relax

Relaxation is slightly different from celebration but on the same playing field. We use the word 'relaxation' to imply anything that helps us to rest, unwind and regenerate on a daily basis, either alone or in the company of other people.

Relaxation is a very personal thing – some people find watching a scary movie relaxing [not us!], others use breathing exercises to ward off tension, how about a soothing massage, a walk in the park – there are a million and one different ways to relax. Naturally a degree of realism is called for – there is more to relaxation than lying on a tropical beach once a year. We encourage you to find ways to relax that suit your body, your mind and your lifestyle. When you are genuinely relaxed, everything in life becomes easier. Now you can relax, celebrate and creatively enjoy the 7th Enrichment Experience Action Area.

The 7th Enrichment Experience Action Area

This is your chance to explore your creative nature, for tasking yourself and enjoying the process of completing a project. You can look at your relationships with children, your ability to engage playfully, to celebrate and to relax. Choose whichever Actions feel right for you.

ACTION A: Questions & answers – your motivating letter

Write yourself a personal letter [Dear Me . . . and the date] in which you answer one or more of the following questions.

Are you making the most of your inbuilt creativity and bringing your projects to fruition?

Do you value your interactions with children and engage playfully with youngsters?

When it comes to celebration and relaxation, what activities best serve your well-being?

Have your answers to any of these questions highlighted the benefit of spending more time on being creative, or of giving 100% to your creative projects when you are engaged in them? What about finishing them to your satisfaction? Perhaps you realise the value of connecting with the playfulness of children, having a cause for celebration or relaxation? Write a few words about any changes you intend to make over the next few months that involve completing projects, playing with children, celebration and relaxation.

Headline your final paragraph with the words "Glad to be alive." Choose three things, related in some way to the 7th Enrichment, that 'make your heart sing'. For instance, the amazing sense of achievement when you finish a creative project, the joy of having fun with children, or maybe you have a friend who gives a super-relaxing massage. An easy way to do this is to finish the sentence: "I'm glad that ……..''

Put your completed letter in an envelope [preferably white] and place it in the west of your home. The significance of this direction will become apparent in ACTION B. From time to time when you feel the need, re-visit your letter and update it.

ACTION B: Create an inspiring environment

The west of your property is considered a good place to celebrate the completion of your creative projects, and to relax with the family around an open hearth – maybe even watch some TV together. In ancient China this area was considered the domain of the passionate and unpredictable white tiger, so wacky and fun could describe your approach.

Don't let clutter stifle your creativity

Is anything cluttering up the areas of your property where you are at your most creative? In addition, pay attention to the west of your home or the west of your living room and you will know intuitively if you need to have a big tidy up.

Ideally remove every single item from the areas you have identified and then replace only those items that are really necessary. Part of your 'clean-start' in the west could be to create a 'clean-look' by painting the walls white [as in the 6th Enrichment] – symbolically a blank canvas for your creativity to flourish; metallic colours and finishes are also well suited.

Focus Features – placing on purpose – physical reminders

Here are some ideas for the west or wherever you chose to honour the 7th Enrichment. They are not prescriptive, just do what feels good for you, only one or two things at a time:

- Position a working metallic clock, a motion ornament or piece of metal sculpture on the mantelpiece or wall symbolising creativity in action.

- Think of the west as an area for your own harvest festival and use this idea to determine your décor.

- Position your stereo system here and play suitable music – arousing, relaxing, fun – depending on the mood you are trying to create.

- Position your TV here and watch 'healthy-for-your-mind' programmes, avoiding those that portray gratuitous violence or constant family bickering and disputes.

- Stand in the west and sing at the top of your voice – chanting on one note is fine.

- Place 'happy family' photographs in a metal frame on the wall or mantelpiece.

- Display paintings, drawings or photographs that you or a family member have created. Children's paintings look really good if you give them a border mount. Change your display from time to time.

- Buy a really comfortable couch which ensures your seating position is good for your back and enjoy that relaxing feeling at the end of the day.

- If you want to boost your creativity, take a piece of white paper and, using a silver or gold pen, write down what you are actually going to do, date it and seal in a white envelope. Place the envelope on a metal plate or bowl, if appropriate to your selected display area. Open it in three months and note what has changed in your life.

ACTION C: What's the real secret?

There is a simple truth behind being successfully creative and it is contained in our exercise called 'What's the Real Secret?'. We have borrowed it from an ancient wisdom teaching and added just a few contemporary ideas, however the secret remains exactly the same!

First take a sheet of white paper – folio or A4.

Fold it in half; fold it in half again; fold it in half a third time.

You now have a small 'card' which is an eighth the size of the original sheet.

[1] Write on the front of the card the following words: Once upon a time there was a great Teacher whom people looked upon with favour and admiration. The Teacher was successful, content, serene and had great wisdom. One day an aspiring student, wishing to become like the Teacher, decided to ask for the 'secret' of success. "Oh great Teacher, I wish to become like you, please tell me your secret." "Happily" replied the Teacher, "every day I study and observe the world."

[2] Open the card up so it is a quarter the size of the original sheet and write the following words 'landscape' across both 'pages': "Yes, oh Teacher, I know that I need to study hard and observe the world. But what is your secret?" "Before I embark on a course of action, I think clearly about what I am trying to achieve. I acknowledge my motives. I use all my senses. I listen to the views of others. I try not to make false assumptions. I allow time to work things out. I approach my task in a positive way", replied the smiling Teacher.

[3] Open the card up so it is half the size of the original sheet and write the following words 'portrait' down the page: "Yes, great Teacher, even these things I know. But tell me, please, what is your secret?" "I am organised and I know what I want. I know where I am going and why. I plan what I do. I continue to learn and improve my skills. I treat my body and mind with respect. I enjoy my time. I try to find ways to give a little bit extra every day." "All these things I acknowledge. What I want to know, great Teacher,

is your real secret?" The wise Teacher was impressed that the student understood there was something more to learn, "Then I will tell you ……..''

[4] Open the page up to its full size and write the following words landscape across the middle in large CAPITAL LETTERS: "I ACTUALLY DO THOSE THINGS THAT OTHER PEOPLE ONLY TALK ABOUT"

[5] Re-fold the paper and then read your leaflet slowly, unfolding as you go. The punch line is a gift for overcoming procrastination. Re-read your card whenever you feel stuck in a rut. Perhaps make a card for anyone you think might benefit from this inspiration [without being offended]. The card also makes a good workshop motivation tool.

ACTION D: Make a difference – change something

How are creativity, children, celebration and relaxation going to feature in your life in future? Are you ready for a practical commitment to do something differently which ensures you achieve your creative goals? The message of the 7th Enrichment Experience is to believe in yourself – in your power to create and to bring that creation to a successful stage where you can celebrate and rejoice.

THE 8th ENRICHMENT EXPERIENCE

Sanctuary; humanitarian and spiritual inquiry; belief; faith; reflection; meditation; solitude; meaning and purpose; mortality; moral values and personal integrity; thanksgiving. *"My country is the world and my religion is to do good."* Thomas Paine 1737-1809.

The constituents of the 8th Enrichment Experience embrace our innermost thoughts and beliefs, the propensity for trying to make sense of our humanity, our need for meaning and purpose including – for some people – religious faith, the moral values and ethics that we choose to live by and our opportunities to be grateful and give thanks. Being fully aware of what it is we actually believe, alongside taking personal responsibility for the consequences of such beliefs, are both vital factors for initiating change in the way we live.

The contemplative side of human nature – that part of us which seeks to understand our place in the universe – is both a personal and a cultural phenomenon. As children, we are generally raised in the doctrines and beliefs of our parents, relatives and the community; although later in adolescence and adulthood, we may choose to question those beliefs and even break free from them.

Your choice of beliefs

In our exploration of the 8th Enrichment we do not intend to discuss the merits or otherwise of specific religious, atheistic or scientific belief systems. However, we do invite you to be fully aware of your choices in this regard and how you personally experience the marvellous mystery that is life on earth. In particular, we can all find opportunities to give thanks for the gift of consciousness through which we manifest our 'reality' and how the wise use of this gift brings meaning and fulfilment to our lives.

The following edited extract from the Rockefeller Center inscription, New York, gives an indication of the sort of beliefs you might like to consider.

> ➤ I believe in the supreme worth of the individual and in his right to life, liberty and the pursuit of happiness.

> ➤ I believe every right implies a responsibility; every opportunity, an obligation; every possession, a duty.

> ➤ I believe … that character, not wealth or power or position, is of supreme worth.

> ➤ I believe that the rendering of useful service is the common duty of humankind and only in the purifying fire of sacrifice is the dross of selfishness consumed and the greatness of the human soul set free.

> ➤ I believe that love is the greatest thing in the world; that it alone can overcome hate; that right can and will triumph over might.

Reflection and self-examination

"The life which is not examined is not worth living" is a challenging statement attributed to Plato. Reading it certainly makes for a slightly uncomfortable feeling which may spur us on to contemplate what it is about our lives that is 'worth living'. Fortuitously, every single human being has within them the potential for worthwhile living. The 8th Enrichment Experience helps us to uncover our unique expression of that potential. We can choose to think through our lives alone in solitude or contemplate and discuss issues in company, or a mixture of both.

J Neville Ward urges us to *"find ways of securing occasions for solitude and thought"*.

Solitude

First consider the delight of solitude: it is a rejuvenating state, not to be confused with loneliness. Unlike loneliness which implies a sad quality, we can actively choose solitude as a time for personal space and inner reflection. Wordsworth, in his famous poem 'Daffodils', describes 'the bliss of solitude' as experienced by 'his inward eye'. This idea of knowing inner bliss through solitary reflection is something we can all aspire to and discover through direct personal experience. Keeping the silence, meditation, call it what you will, offers a channel to our innermost essence and satisfies our hunger for deeper meaning – some would say a spiritual connection to the universal wisdom of the divine.

Meditation

Today many people in America and Europe practice meditation – traditionally a concept of Asian and Far Eastern cultures. Various techniques can be employed such as concentrating on the breath or having single-point focus on a mantra or simply observing thoughts as they arise and letting them go, rather than indulging them. We give more detail in Appendix D: Mindfulness practice, and 'Thoughts – let them go!' in the 8th Enrichment Action Area below.

One good reason to meditate is to free ourselves from attachment and desire – the root causes of our own suffering. Being immersed in the meditative state is an experience beyond the ideas and concepts we generally hold and describe to others using words and images – you have to 'experience' it for yourself.

The wise teacher Krishnamurti proposes that even using the label 'experience' is difficult in that experiences are necessarily in the past and meditation is in the present moment. He regards meditation as the process of understanding one's own mind by watching it – paying attention to what your mind does and asking 'who it is whose actually observing the thoughts?'.

You can meditate by whatever means works for you – a formal system doesn't necessarily suit everyone. It is, however, accepted that understanding your mind – complete realisation of the truth of your existence – defies description. You will know it when you feel it.

The science of calming the mind

Several scientific studies of people who meditate regularly have shown changes in their brain activity as recorded on EEG [Electro Encephalo Graph] brain scanning equipment. Interestingly changes in the physical and biochemical bodily functions of practiced meditators have also been recorded. It is good to know that if we choose to meditate regularly, we can have a positive influence on our metabolism, heart rate, respiration, blood pressure and brain chemistry.

Meditation starts with calming the mind as HH The Dalai Lama explains in The True Expression of Non-violence is Compassion: *"Unless our minds are stable and calm, no matter how comfortable our physical conditions may be, they will give us no pleasure. Therefore, the key to a happy life, now and in the future, is to develop a happy mind"*.

There are of course different ways to address this apparent human need to understand our place in the universe and our own mortality – whether or not we believe in a spiritual existence beyond this world. Participating in the 8th Enrichment Experience acts as a personal prompt for those of us who wish to engage in humanitarian spiritual inquiry, either alone or in communion with like-minded people.

A word about 'spiritual shopping'

When people set about changing their lives, for a small minority, there can be a strange fascination with all things 'spiritual', including so-called New Age 'wisdom'. Exploring their faith and beliefs can lead to over-the-top 'spiritual shopping', sometimes at a fairly shallow level. Of course, if you are not already sure of your belief system, we suggest that you 'shop around' in order to learn about different approaches and to find the one that resonates with you.

Ideally your belief system will be open to rational inquiry based on evidence; for example, we believe that the fossil record validates the theory of evolution wherein homo sapiens is a highly-evolved sentient being endowed with consciousness. Believing in evolution in no way diminishes total awe for the wonders of our planet and the universe with its trillions of stars and galaxies almost beyond imagination.

While you are considering your creed and ethics, it is sensible to keep an eye on how your journey is progressing, just in case you are falling into the spiritual shopping trap. In extreme cases, spiritual shopping can lead to a needy materialistic-type attachment to certain gurus, teachings or purchases. The chronic proliferation of Buddha statues in the homes and gardens of people who do not even bother to find out anything about the Buddha or the Dharma [the teachings], is testament to this fad. The same goes for Ganesh, the Hindu deity with distinctive elephant head and human body. Ganesh symbolises intellect and wisdom in the arts and sciences, and the removal of obstacles. Ganesh is especially revered at the beginning of rituals. Now his statue too is becoming a designer item.

If we are going to align ourselves with a particular belief system or teacher or set of ethics, then we will only do them and ourselves justice by 'walking the talk' and understanding what it is that we have signed up to. The same goes if we decide to take an eclectic mix-and-match approach, we need to be aware of the principles that we are using as guidance because whatever we chose to believe will have an influence on how our lives unfold.

Have a reality check on the meaning of life

Which ideologies do you hold, if any, to make sense of your existence and the meaning of life? In particular, have you ever considered the nature of 'your reality'? Is it actually an illusion or is it the ultimate truth? How is your idea of what constitutes reality reflected in the way you live your life? Is your happiness and well-being somehow linked to this idea?

Getting to grips with reality is a 'real' challenge. Most of our thoughts and actions stem from a belief in some kind of 'reality', so it is important to know what we 'really' mean. By questioning ourselves we can reveal some of our underlying beliefs concerning reality which undoubtedly influence our subsequent attitudes, actions and experiences. If you want to explore this reality thread further, please see Appendix K where the subject is discussed in greater detail.

We can make a choice, every single day, either to create 'a reality' that looks no further than our problems or to action 'the reality of leading a meaningful life'. We can manifest joy and gladness whenever possible and allow our personal expressive nature to shine through, radiating the means to serve and love other people.

'Being happy' – a flourishing life

Philosophers talk about 'flourishing' to describe a life well-lived. We can equate this well-lived life as 'being happy', allowing for the fact that there will always be some tough times when calm composure is the best we can do. So we could say our purpose is 'to be happy' and to help others by spreading this happiness. We can make our life journey more purposeful by mindfully focusing on being as helpful as possible to ourselves and to others, always allowing our innate happiness to shine forth. Easier said than done!

Even when there are no obvious physical or emotional hardships in sight, some people find happiness a difficult state to achieve. In order to enjoy 'a happy life', you need to discover exactly what fulfils you personally – body, mind and spirit. Your innate capacity 'to be happy' is inside you all the time. To liberate your happiness state, you can learn to release any emotional bonds or damaging attitudes you may unwittingly have put in place – things you have chosen, often subconsciously, that sabotage your flourishing nature. So give yourself time and space to develop a flourishing happiness habit – on purpose – then spread it around!

Obviously here we are talking about 'appropriate happiness' which also acknowledges 'appropriate sadness' – the complementary opposites that motivate our lives to a greater or lesser extent. There will always be times when we experience unavoidable suffering through grief, sadness and pain. This cycle of being happy and suffering is 'a reality' for everyone, therefore we embrace the duality of our existence and determine to see the silver linings whenever possible.

Reflecting on mortality

"I want us to be doing things, prolonging life's duties as much as we can; I want death to find me planting my cabbages, neither worrying about it nor the unfinished gardening." Montaigne.

Today the life expectancy of someone living in the US or UK is higher than it has ever been. Many of us will live well into our 80s and 90s, unless we fall prey to accident or disease. At the other end of the scale are certain African countries where life expectancy has fallen dramatically due to the spread of HIV, civil war, famine and abject poverty.

In 2007 alone, some nine million children died before the age of five worldwide. Clearly there are victims who have little, or no, control over their destinies. While acknowledging this massive and unacceptable inequality of life expectation, the awareness of lifespan we are referring to here is for people who do have choice.

Paradoxically we may find it helpful in our efforts to live life well, if we occasionally reflect on our own mortality – the end of our existence as we know it. There is no denying that death is a fact of life that impacts us all – the death of a loved one, the tragedy of an innocent victim, our view of our own demise – so it would be remiss of us not to address it. The time we have on this earth within our corporal bodies is limited to the years between our birth and our death. This is not intended as a morbid statement, just the truth, for while we freely talk about birth, death is often a subject in denial.

In whatever way we decide to live, one day we will die. How much better, then, to have lived a life in which we tried to make worthwhile contributions to our families and to society, rather than one where we squandered our time on earth in aimless self-indulgence and mediocrity? Have you ever attended the funeral of an elderly person who has lived generously and, far from sombre, found the service to be a celebration for a beautiful life? This is how we too can be remembered, if we choose a life well-lived.

Sadly, there will always be tragic and untimely death due to illness, crime, accident or natural disaster. For those of us who have experience of this, there are no easy answers. However, it is true that our loved ones who have died would not want us to suffer for ever, or even at all. They would like to see us finding some way to come to terms with their death, finding something positive within the tragedy that might include helping others to avoid the same fate. This is often how campaigns and charities come into being, including those for medical research, restorative justice, safer products and practices.

When people we know die, it is often a time of personal reflection. With serene acceptance, we may choose to think about our own mortality; to do this can actually be life enhancing and invigorating. It makes us aware that we have the privilege of this fragile gift of life, so we can honour it in the best ways we know how.

Moral values and tolerance

Most of us intuitively know what is right or wrong, good or bad, virtuous or fatuous, depending on the circumstances. And our personal integrity is bound up in the way we manifest our values in practice. Yet, unless we are signed up to a religious or humanist code of ethics, if asked to state our moral values, we might hesitate. There is no agreed secular standard for ethical values apart from statutory obligations laid down in law. Many of the daily choices and decisions that we make fall outside this legal framework but are, nonetheless, reflective of our moral stance.

In addition to our personal day-to-day morality, there are conversations to be had about the human rights of terrorists, genetically modified species, contemporary medical ethics – including embryonic research, euthanasia, or where to draw the line on cognitive performance enhancement. The philosophical paradox of tolerance is ever with us – this is particularly apt with the rise of extremist terrorist groups. Karl Popper concluded that we are warranted in refusing to tolerate intolerance: *"We should therefore claim, in the name of tolerance, the right not to tolerate the intolerant."*

As you contemplate various aspects of the 8th Enrichment, you may like to consider the nature of your personal integrity and set of values. The elements of your life well-lived could include always being responsible for yourself and for your life choices, trying to practise non-judgemental compassion towards others, giving love and kindness unconditionally, never knowingly doing anything to harm others, not sitting on the side-lines harping criticism but constructively getting involved, being thankful for what is fortunate in your life and, as much as possible, happily enjoying the good times.

An attitude of gratitude

The US public holiday of Thanksgiving in November is a good example of setting aside a special time in which to be grateful for family and friends, and the goodness of the land on which we are privileged to live, wherever we are in the world. But there is no need to restrict our thanksgiving to just once a year. We can be grateful for these blessings every day of our lives.

Perhaps you can think of a way to build a 'thanksgiving' moment or two into your daily schedule? How about starting the day with an attitude of gratitude? First thing in the morning in bed, you could give yourself a big stretch and smile while thinking of some of the things that you have to be grateful for, and the ways in which you can manifest this thanks during the coming day. How lucky you are to be greeting the day with the life force coursing through your amazing physical body.

Here is a lovely quote from M J Ryan about expressing thankfulness: *"Gratitude is like a flashlight. As you shine it on what's right in your life, you experience more satisfaction, connection and fulfilment. All you have to do to experience its effects is turn it on."*

Time to stand and stare

Rush, rush, rush – busy, busy, busy – worry, worry, worry – must be perfect, must be perfect, must be perfect – is this the way we want to live our lives? In the words of the writer William Henry Davies [1870-1940]: *"What is this life, if full of care, we have no time to stand and stare?"*

What sort of things would you like to stand and stare at, or sit and contemplate? Maybe it is just a case of taking some 'me-time' to re-connect with the core of your being so that you get back on track to live the life that is right for you. So many of us today get caught up on a treadmill and forget the reason why we are doing what we are doing.

Here's a little poem that expresses this sentiment:

> *I used to be the hare*
>
> *Raring to go*
>
> *Always quick off the mark*
>
> *Life in the fast lane*
>
> *Everything a rush*
>
> *Now I'm an understudy*
>
> *For the tortoise*
>
> *And I'm learning the part .... slowly yet surely.*

The 8th Enrichment Experience Action Area

Consider this a quiet contemplative Action Area because it is an opportunity to satisfy your hunger for a deeper sense of your existence within the universe – the beauty of the anima mundi. Your inner life can be compared to a secret greenhouse where the seeds of your mind gently germinate before you transplant them into the garden of daily existence to flourish and yield their fruit. Choose from the following suggestions and exercises to enhance your thoughtfulness.

ACTION A: Questions & answers – your motivating letter

Write yourself a personal letter [Dear Me . . . and the date] in which you answer one or more of the following questions:

If asked what your beliefs are, what would you say? Be completely honest here.

Who, or what, do you allow to disturb your peace of mind – including yourself?

Do you have lots of things to be grateful for? Name a few.

Have your answers to any of these questions helped you to see your humanity in a different light? Write a couple of sentences about how you intend to nurture this aspect of your life over the next few weeks and months?

Headline your final paragraph with the words "Glad to be alive." Choose three things, related in some way to the 8th Enrichment, that 'make your heart sing'. For instance, being comfortable with your beliefs and moral principles; being able to see the path of your life purpose? An easy way to do this is to finish the sentence: "I'm glad that ...."

Put your completed letter in an envelope [preferably purple or an earthy colour like brown] and place it in the north east of your home or a designated sacred space if you have one. The significance of this will become apparent in ACTION B.

ACTION B: Create an inspiring environment

The north east of your property is deemed to be a sacred area where you can take time out to be deeply in touch with your consciousness, your ethical beliefs for living a good life and, for some, religious inquiry. In the Hindu tradition, the family shrine room is positioned in the north east, likewise oriental Feng Shui recognised this direction for the purposes of contemplation and meditation. However, we recommend choosing any area of your home that feels right for you.

Clarity of thought or confusion?

Is your 'spiritual' path clear as crystal or is it cluttered with confusion? Take a look in the north east of your home, or another area that feels like a calm 'thinking space', and see what is present there. Are there any clues from the function of the room, the objects and the colours?

Clear away any surplus or inappropriate items. Pay particular attention to 'having too much of a good thing'. For example, one stunning antique or eye-catching picture is helpful, too many and you fail to enjoy even the beauty of one. Clean the floor and walls thoroughly.

Focus Features – placing on purpose – physical reminders

'Keep it simple yet regal' is the message for honouring the 8th Enrichment in the north east of your home, the north east of a suitable room or whichever area feels like a sanctuary. Here are some ideas – only one or two things at a time as appropriate to your particular belief system:

- You can dedicate a suitable place in your home as a sacred space and create an altar/personal shrine here.

- The images and objects that you place on your altar are entirely up to you, depending on your particular beliefs. Only display statues or sacred objects that represent the values and beliefs you have studied and are prepared to live by.

- This can be a good place to position an easy chair and a shelf for books that inspire and connect you to your spiritual nature.

- If you meditate, you can create a special space for your practice with appropriate floor cushions or, if you are elderly or infirm, a suitable chair.

- A vase of fresh violet or lilac coloured flowers, such as lavender, will enliven your 'thinking about thinking' and provide a calming aroma.

- The north east suits the display of one or two prime earth objects – especially auspicious are crystals of amethyst and citrine or nuggets of amber – they can represent thanksgiving for the earth.

- Sacred statues placed in the north east of your garden should always be positioned on a plinth and their symbolic qualities known to you.

ACTION C: Thoughts – let them go!

'Thoughts – let them go' is a basic system for quietening the mind – otherwise known as single-pointed mindfulness meditation. The length of time you spend meditating is entirely your choice – even 5 to 10 minutes a day is beneficial. A few basic instructions:

[1] Make sure you won't be disturbed so pre-plan your session.

[2] Turn off or avoid phones, clocks, distracting noises, bright lights etc.

[3] Be wide awake so choose not to meditate when you are likely to feel sleepy.

[4] Wear loose clothing or at least do not feel restricted in any way by your clothes.

[5] Get into a comfortable position – it is fine to sit in a chair or lie on the floor/couch as long as you are wide awake.

[6] Bring your breathing under conscious control for a few moments to calm your body and mind.

[7] Now begin to focus your mind on just one thing – suggestions:

- your breathing – focus on every 'out breath';
- a sound or mantra – om [aum] or hu are popular, or choose your own sound;
- a simple mental image eg. the sun, a white light, a cross, an ankh, a lotus flower, an empty vessel, anything that feels right for you.

[8] As you attempt to meditate in this way, you will find that other thoughts come to you. It is quite normal for thoughts to come in, so it is important you don't feel you are 'failing' at meditation. Every time you find yourself dwelling on new thoughts, just label them 'thoughts', let them go and return to your focus – your out breath or mantra or special image. Remember – 'thoughts

need attention to survive' – so do not give them your attention!

Using single-pointed mindfulness, you can train your mind to give 100% attention to things that really matter and refuse to allow 'your chattering mind' to take over. After a while, you will find that the process of 'letting go of your thoughts' becomes a natural habit. Many people find that the time they spend meditating is more than paid back during the working day because somehow they seem to work smarter.

ACTION D: Make a difference – change something

What sort of things could you do to enhance your moral welfare and the contemplative side of life? Your commitment to the 8th Enrichment recognises the choices you make to uphold your beliefs and values – choices that are conducive to living with integrity, cultivating calmness and being of service to others. Try to make time, as often as is practical, to think about your reasons to be grateful and ways to encourage the expression of your inbuilt happy nature.

Things I'm learning to be . . .

calm ~ content ~ connected ~ wise ~ wonderful ~ well ~ positive ~ peaceful ~ precious ~ fearless ~ forgiving ~ free

THE 9th ENRICHMENT EXPERIENCE

Confidence and self-esteem; empowerment; expression; inspiration; motivation; recognition; significance; fame; shining your light; experiencing life to the full. *"Experience is not what happens to you. It is what you do with what happens to you."* Aldous Huxley.

Our sense of self – the ego – and how we express ourselves as we experience the world, are the prime focus of the 9th Enrichment. And doing this spot of navel gazing is far from selfish. The theory is that working on personal self-respect and our view of our self, informs the way we behave towards others. We learn to unlock our potential for being nicer, kinder and happier people to the benefit of all.

Describing ego

There are many words to describe the condition of self – which ones resonate with you? Take a look at the following descriptive words in alphabetical order. Some are pleasant, some neutral, some not so pleasant. Talk yourself through them and discover if some of these words have special significance for you. If so, it may help you to explore why?

Self-aggrandisement ~ self-approval ~ self-assertive ~ self-assured ~ self-aware ~ self-confident ~ self-controlled ~ self-conscious ~ self-deception ~ self-denial ~ self-development ~ self-discipline ~ self-effacement ~ self-empowerment ~ self-esteem ~ self-expression ~ self-help ~ self-image ~ self-important ~ self-improvement ~ selfish ~ selfless ~ self-opinionated ~ self-pity ~ self-possessed ~ self-realisation ~ self-regard ~ self-reliant ~ self-reproach ~ self-respect ~ self-restraint

~ self-righteous ~ self-sabotage ~ self-sacrifice ~ self-satisfied ~ self-sufficient ~ self-willed ~ self-worth.

Knowing your 'ego-type' can help you, especially if you decide to challenge the ideas you currently hold about your ability to perform and live life to the full. In this context, how do you regard self-esteem? There is a lot of talk these days about problems associated with having 'low or poor self-esteem' – we need to be clear what this actually means.

Self-esteem – finding the happy medium

What exactly are we talking about when we refer to self-esteem? For the purposes of the 9th Enrichment, we are talking about 'good' self-esteem as meaning healthy self-respect and empowerment.

Your self-esteem is linked to how you feel about what you believe other people think or say about you, which is fine if you believe that their opinions and comments are fair and reasonable. This is, of course, not always the case. Two examples of rare extremes help to illustrate the importance of maintaining healthy self-esteem.

On the one hand, there is self-aggrandisement – the result of people putting someone on a pedestal – think charlatan cult leaders, power-crazed politicians or autocratic despots. High self-esteem without moral responsibility has given us tyrants and dictators such as Hitler, Stalin, Pol Pot and Pinochet.

On the other hand, there is the extreme low self-esteem of mental torment – often the result of emotional bullying that may include unjust or unfounded reputation bashing. In tragic cases, the latter has led to victims becoming severely depressed and possibly even suicidal. NB. If you are being bullied or have mental health problems, please consult a qualified professional. The 9th Enrichment

Experience is not a substitute for appropriate care or treatment.

When it comes to self-esteem, finding a happy medium is key. As you probably realise, your present level of self-esteem, and all manner of associated characteristics, is entwined with a great many factors. It would be misguided to suggest that you can simply change your feelings about yourself overnight – although you might like to try. However, over time with practice, you most certainly can.

Confidence in action

Typically, there are many of us who would just like to feel a bit better about ourselves, particularly when we encounter life's difficulties. Rather than seeking approval from others, which may be a carry-over from childhood [with-holding of parental approval being a crucial factor for some of us], you could dare to have confidence in your ability to show the world the person you aspire to be – right here and right now.

In order to boost your confidence, you could start by 'thinking from outside' – pretend you are observing yourself. You may see that 'approval of yourself', which underpins your confidence, need not depend on the opinions you think other people may have about you. [We are assuming here that you are not behaving in a way that harms others]. So there is nothing to lose if you jettison your fears and worries about what other people may think and concentrate instead on approving of yourself as a personable human being.

With confidence, and the psychological security that this brings, you can build a 'can-do' attitude which we discussed in Chapter 8 [Part 1]. Having a 'can-do and will-do' attitude makes such a difference as to how we express ourselves and how we experience life. We no longer need to seek approval, or feel guilty about not living up to someone else's expectations, to feel confident that our lives are worthwhile.

Can't or won't?

The old saying "there's no such word as can't" is tremendously helpful when you are trying to establish a healthy confident frame of mind. Next time you find yourself saying "I can't ……..", substitute "I don't want to …….." or "I won't ……..", then see how the statement feels. You might be empowered to change the 'can't mentality' to something more positive. When duty calls and you sigh "I have to ……..", substitute "I'd like to …….." and smile to yourself.

Having confidence in your innate ability to be sensitive, responsive, compassionate and open to your own well-being ultimately benefits everyone. You start by opening up to the process of 'unlearning' any unhelpful ingrained habits and you come to appreciate your place in this extra-ordinary mystery which is life on earth. Hey presto – confidence.

In control or being controlled?

Here's a useful affirmation: *"Today my achievements can be many if I choose not to waste my precious time anguishing over people or situations I cannot control."* Alongside self-confidence, there is another feature of the 9th Enrichment Experience which can have a profound impact on our lives – that of 'control'. Sometimes, through no apparent fault of your own, you may find yourself in circumstances where you have little or no control over the presenting situation – although at a subliminal level you may have attracted some of its elements.

By way of example, you may feel anxious and stressed at work because your boss is being impossible, or during a family dispute where two of your relatives have fallen out and are pulling you into the argument. Even though the situation is not of your making, you are involved and yet not in control. You can maintain your self-respect, by seeing the reality of where the control actually lies.

If you do find yourself in such a 'controlled' environment, your best bet is to accept 'what is' and decide purposefully on a course of action or non-action, being as diplomatic as possible, but also being true to yourself. Always try to be resourceful and see the possibilities that may exist within a situation, including avoidance, when you are currently powerless to change the control.

On the other hand, when 'the control', or partial control, for a particular situation is yours, you can take responsibility for what happens next. The 9th Enrichment Experience asks you to openly acknowledge your character strengths and weaknesses, so you can empower yourself to take control of your decisions, thereby creating the life you need to flourish. In the words of Inglehart: *"Ultimately, the most important determinant of happiness is the extent to which people have free choice in how to live their lives"*. By understanding the extent to which you have control, and therefore responsibility, you can undoubtedly make better choices.

Recognition – being significant

Taking a slightly different angle as to how we see ourselves, consider whether or not you feel it is important to be acknowledged and recognised? One of the criteria reported by psychologists as being a key ingredient for a contented and happy life is recognition from others which they term 'significance'. William James [referred to as 'The Father of American Psychology] wrote in the late 1800s:

"The deepest principle in human nature is the craving to be appreciated."

Being significant and appreciated means to be visible, to be wanted, to be recognised and respected by other people. For most of us, this means having a decent reputation among our friends and family, work colleagues and leisure buddies. Our reputation generally stems from our actions, including speech, writing, and visual presentation, and what others say about us – true or false. If false, we may decide to take steps to refute the untruth.

Having a healthy regard for fairness and feeling significant for the right reasons both play an important part in your ability to express yourself. Conversely, caring too much about your reputation and desperately seeking recognition, is unhelpful. The best practice is always to find a balance.

For the purpose of engaging in the 9th Enrichment Experience, it helps to adopt a lifestyle that allows you to be true to yourself, while being socially engaged with people who recognise and appreciate the significance of your unique contribution. And when you need a challenge, you could try stepping out of your comfort zone and see what being insignificant or unrecognised feels like. It is actually a great test of unpretentiousness and humility.

Fame and celebrity

Taking the idea of recognition a step further, what about today's obsession with fame and celebrity? For some people recognition – being significant – takes on a whole new meaning. These are people who, for whatever reason, attract fame either intentionally or coincidentally – politicians, academics, entrepreneurs, sports champions, musicians, actors, artists, writers, models, socialites and broadcasters.

Fame, as we all know, is a double-edged sword – so be careful what you wish for. Losing valued privacy is one of the first challenges of fame, along with the very real threat to famous individuals of being targeted by criminal extortionists or people with mental health issues.

Seeking fame seems to have reached epidemic proportions in recent years. The 21st century has opened with a litany of reality TV shows preying on the desire for superstardom. These are several types including programmes that give people with real skills, which they have worked hard to develop, the opportunity to reach a wider audience and possibly find a sponsor. But for every 'success' there will be many disappointments. Other shows take a diverse group of volunteers and place them in extreme environments to see how they cope. The worst offenders are shows that promise people with undeveloped or infamous talent, the chance for notoriety as they wash their dirty linen in public.

When recognition from others becomes a media circus, it is time to ask what sort of values we are putting forward for our children and grandchildren to aspire to? Fame at any price is a dangerous commodity. Thankfully there are still those people worthy of being role models who earn their reputation through skill and hard work. Let us acknowledge and emulate the world's conscientious philanthropists who use their fame to help others through a variety of measures including financial sponsorship, clean water and food aid, providing educational resources, medical interventions, lobbying governments and championing peace.

Inspiration and motivation

The challenge of the 9th Enrichment is to fire ourselves up and get out there to experience the world in all its mayhem and all its glory. What do we need for this task? We need to have good intentions. We need discrimination. We need to be practical and in it for the long-term. We need inspiration and motivation.

Where do we find inspiration and motivation? Inside and outside. We can draw these qualities from within by following our intuition, and then by planning practical ways to manifest our hopes and dreams. Looking outside, we can find people whom we admire and respect and emulate them as our role models. We can find projects to fit with our ideas of progress and involve ourselves wholeheartedly in them.

We can find inspiration from the humblest of people and motivation from the tallest of mountains. We can roll a dice, search the internet and use our imagination. We can be galvanised into action by Hannibal's advice: *"We will either find a way or we will make one."*

Shine brightly

Metaphorically the 9th Enrichment Experience honours the active element of fire which occurs naturally in our homes as sunshine – we are en<u>light</u>ened as to the immense possibilities of using our skills and talents wisely with warmth and compassion. Best of all, if we are altruistic, this can be a pay-it-forward experience – our inspired, motivated selves provide the fire and inspiration for others to branch out and excel. *"If you are lucky enough to find a way of life you love, you have to find the courage to live it."* John Irving.

The 9th Enrichment Experience Action Area

Inspiration and motivation are key elements of the following suggestions and exercises. They can help you discover what, if anything, you might like to change in order to bolster your self-respect and confidence so you find suitable outlets for your talents and brightness. Choose the actions that resonate with you, disregard the others.

ACTION A: Questions & answers – your motivating letter

Write yourself a personal letter [Dear Me . . . and the date] in which you answer one or more of the following questions:

How well do you know yourself – do you see yourself as insecure or as confident in your ability to achieve whatever you set your mind to?

Do you care too much about what you think other people may think about you?

Thinking about untried opportunities for using your talents and skills what, if anything, is holding you back?

Do your answers highlight areas where a slight shift in the way you see yourself, your attitude or frame of mind, could make a difference to your self-expression, motivation and ultimately your experiences?

As you write your letter, you may find you are having interesting thoughts about the way you intend to immerse yourself in various experiences over the next few years. Have any of your answers highlighted areas where you could develop your self-confidence and allow yourself to do things that, in the past, may have appeared daunting and scary? Maybe write a few words about how you intend to 'fire yourself up' and realistically initiate change by using the 9th Enrichment know-how to enhance your well-being. Be constructive so your letter expresses positive intentions.

Headline your final paragraph with the words "Glad to be alive." Choose three things, related in some way to the 9th Enrichment, that 'make your heart sing'. For instance, do you feel inspired to approve of yourself and determined to live life to the full? Are there things that you can do to inspire others? An easy way to do this is to finish the sentence: "I'm glad that ……….."

Seal your letter in a red envelope and date the back. Place it in the south of your home or the south of the room you spend most time in. Open it in one year's time. See how you have progressed. If you like the result, then please repeat annually. The significance of the southern placement will become apparent in ACTION B.

ACTION B: Create an inspiring environment

You can fire yourself up for approval and action by paying attention to the south of your property or the southern aspect of your main living room or the room in which you spend most time. In Feng Shui these areas are said to represent fire energy which generates motivation, action and expansion for your life – the expression of the sunny side of your nature. As we have already implied, inspiration, self-esteem, personal expression, fame and recognition are all part and parcel of your fire nature.

If you think about it, the sun's rays are at their most intense in the southern parts of your home, giving a certain feel-good factor to these areas. These are the places to be when you need a boost to your self-confidence, to garner inspiration or to experience the warm glow that confirms your intention to engage fully with the world.

How can you tell if there is a blockage to your fire nature? Well you are quite likely to feel trapped, caged, frustrated by a lack of light and open air, unable to spread your wings. Fortunately, there are several things you can do to release yourself and learn to fly again with majestic purpose.

Clearing the areas where inspiration dwells

If your fire area is cluttered, your life could be stale and uninteresting, so take a look around and note what you see – the décor, the furniture, the objects and the pictures are all pertinent. If there are too many symbols of the water element in the south – represented by glass, black, blue and of course water itself, then you may be putting out your fire even before you get going! Ideally remove everything that is portable and then replace only those items that inspire you.

Focus Features – placing on purpose – physical reminders

Here are some ideas to honour the 9th Enrichment in the south of your home or the south of a suitable room. Undertake one or two things at a time, to remind you to feel confident, motivated and ready for wonderful experiences:

- Make sure the south is always well illuminated. If there is no natural light available here [that is, no windows or glass doors because you live in adjoined property], ensure artificial lights are bright and attractive.

- The south is a good place to honour your self-expression by lighting a scented candle. Always be fire safety conscious with candles and remember that they deplete oxygen in a room, so burn sparingly.

- If you enjoy the smell of incense or essential oils [using an oil burner], try frankincense, sandalwood or citronella – they all help to get you going. However, do not burn incense in small rooms without ventilation.

- If your fireplace happens to be in the south, then fire is already a dominant feature. Symbolically sunlight is even stronger for radiating the heat and light of self-expression. Think 'appropriate warmth' and 'functional light' rather than 'dazzling inferno' with its attendant ash-laden burn out which could signify you are doing too much and need to slow down.

- Symbolise the warmth of the sun by using splashes of red and orange to energise yourself into action – you can paint a wall, display a sunny or red fruit picture, accessorise in red depending on the room's function – chair covers, cushions, tablecloths, ornaments etc.

- Be inspired by a vase of fresh flowers or a thriving pot plant – sunflowers, carnations, tulips, chrysanthemums, red geraniums – plants that suggest active blooming.

- Hang a crystal on a silver thread in a southern window. Enjoy the radiating mini-rainbows that will show up on your walls and floors if they are plain white or of pale colour. From a clear-cut crystal, all the colours of the rainbow are experienced. Use this visual image as a metaphor for your own crystal potential being expressed in a multitude of amazing and colourful ways.

- When the sun is shining through your crystal stand in front of it, close your eyes [essential otherwise you may damage them], and feel the beam directed onto the middle of your brow – your 'third eye'. Metaphorically, think how to use this illuminating energy to further your personal development and capability to inspire others.

ACTION C: Fast forward 10 years to view your achievements

This exercise is a smart way to focus the mind on what you would really like to action and accomplish, especially if you are stuck or unsure about which way to go in life. Rather than thinking about what you might be doing this year, next year, in 3 years etc., you are going to mentally leap 10 years into the future and 'look back' on what you have been doing for the past decade.

You may well find that this 'look back' method is a more constructive way to sort out what you really want, than merely dream-wishing for the future. Once you get into this backward vision, you can be quite realistic about which tasks and actions will create the future you desire – then you need to plan them into your daily regime. This is quite a good exercise to do with a close friend. Please read through all the instructions first before starting the mind focus part.

- Adopt a comfortable sitting position and have pen and paper ready in front of you.

- Close your eyes and bring your breathing into your conscious mind. Get a comfortable rhythm going for a minute or two.

- Now 'fast forward' 10 years in your mind. If you are 25 pretend you are 35, if you are 30 be 40, if you are 52 pretend you are 62 and so on.

- Looking back over the decade you have just lived through, reflect on some personal questions along the lines: What would I like to have accomplished? What have I accomplished? What would I like to have enjoyed? What have I enjoyed? What would I like to have tried that's new? What have I tried that's new? Who would I like to have known better? Who have I got to know better? Who would I like to have met? Who did I meet? Where would I like to have been? Where did I go? What changes would I like to have made? What changes did I make? Have I wasted my last 10 years? Have I used my 10 years to the full?

- Still in the mindset of being 10 years older looking back, open your eyes and write down some of the things you 'have done' in the past decade. This is an

entirely personal exercise so the examples below are meant purely for illustration:
   I overcame my shyness
   I got to know my family better
   I moved in with a new partner
   I ditched the processed rubbish and ate proper food
   I took up a sport …..
   I took up a new hobby …..
   I changed my job and now I'm working as a …..
   I do voluntary work for …..
   I've travelled to some interesting places, including …
   I got a lovely pet ….. to care for
   I did several things that gave me a sense of achievement including …..

- You can return to your '10 years looking back' notes at any time – tick off the things you are actually doing and add new things as appropriate. You can even make a display sheet for your notice board if you like. Remember to pace yourself and enjoy doing the small things day-by-day – that is all part of the plan.

Native American Indians have a wonderful ethos for handling the future: *"there should be no worry – just peace – because there is a plan, even it you cannot see it. Wisdom is not in the searching but in the living each day with a good heart and a good mind. Use your intuition and give thanks, then peace will reign"*.

The fact is, if you don't make a start now, in 10 years' time you may not have involved yourself in any of the things that are there for the taking. Nobody else is going to come knocking on your door and say 'today you are going to try this, or start that, or meet so and so . . .' but you can. You can knock on your own inner door, unlock the will to make choices-for-change and go for it. Rather than dreaming the impossible dream, go for 'realising the possible – plus a bit' and see yourself doing it.

ACTION D: Make a difference – change something

This is your chance to make a commitment to change something for the better. Whatever you decide to do, make sure it is in tune with the essence of the 9th Enrichment which requires total awareness of your personal character, your attitudes and your ability to shine in whatever sphere feels right for the full development of your talents and skills. However insignificant your contribution may seem to you right now, it is important to believe you can make a difference – because you can.

Your goal is the journey that enables you to enhance the way you feel about yourself and how you approach, motivate and experience your life. On this journey you can learn to act for the benefit of everyone with whom you come into contact, directly and indirectly. Your reward will be a full and flourishing life. *"Life shrinks or expands in proportion to one's courage."* Anais Nin.

SUSTAINING AN ENRICHED WAY OF LIFE

"Genuine happiness can only be achieved when we transform our way of life from the unthinking pursuit of pleasure to one committed to enriching our inner lives, when we focus on 'being more' rather than simply having more." Daisaku Ikeda.

The Habitat Affect in daily action

Maintaining healthy thinking, wise choices and appropriate enrichment actions on a continuing basis requires positive commitment. This is where your personally devised Habitat Affect comes into play as a daily consistent reminder of your intentions and aspirations.

Each of the 9 Enrichments in Part 2 included an 'ACTION B: Create an inspiring environment for Habitat Affect benefits'. You are encouraged to clear the clutter and then introduce personal Focus Features – physically making changes to chosen areas of your home or workplace environment. Your Focus Features, as already emphasised, act as powerful cues for you to honour the various aspects of your life. They act as significant objective prompts for the choices you make today – and every single day of your life – these are the choices that create your future.

Focus Features summary for your home

Here we give a brief recap of the Focus Features previously recommended in some detail for each of the 9 Enrichment areas. Our summary guide below is organised around the compass directions and symbols associated with the 5 elements. For graphic illustration see Appendix

L: Compass and element chart and Appendix M: The 5 Elements.

Although not essential, if you have drawn an outline plan of your home as mentioned in Chapter 2 [Part 1], you can refer to it again. If you haven't already drawn a plan and feel it would be helpful, draw one now with the windows, doors and compass directions marked on.

You can view your home plan alongside Appendix L and Appendix M plus this Focus Feature summary for each enrichment or, for greater detail, refer back to the 9 individual ACTION B recommendations.

The 1st Enrichment: work; career; vocation; volunteering; using skills; releasing hidden potential; consolidation of ideas; planning; hibernation; the seed waiting in the ground. NORTH – WATER.

Place glass objects and water symbols here. Blue and black are favourable colours. It is a good place to display any work-related items, certificates or trophies. An ornamental tortoise can help you to remember the story of the hare and the tortoise and who won the race! The north represents the consolidation of your efforts and allows you to hibernate by taking a step aside to think about your occupation and work/life balance; perhaps preparing to sow the seeds for change. A place to appreciate the effort you put into work and the opportunities it presents for using your talents and skills, possibly in a volunteering capacity if you have time.

The 2nd Enrichment: personal relationship; love; romance; sexual intimacy; compromise; companionship; the joy of sharing; being contently single; looking for a like-minded soulmate. SOUTH WEST – EARTH.

Make a special place where you display a photograph of yourself and your partner happily together. Alternatively, if you are looking for romance, then a romantic picture or piece of sculpture can energise this aspect of your life. You can also position a piece of rose quartz here or hang a heart-shaped crystal in a south west window. Flowers which symbolise love and romance [roses, peonies, pink carnations, yellow blooms], can be placed in the south west, as can any other personal objects that 'do it for you'. How about a pair of love spoons or a pair of anything that symbolises love and romance? Keep the south west well lit – a heart-shaped candle – a beautiful lamp. Write down your wishes for a loving relationship or copy a love poem and put it in your relationship area – be careful what you wish for!

The 3rd Enrichment: life-long learning; curiosity; engaging new ideas; personal growth; respect for parents, ancestors, elders, teachers, coaches and leaders; initiation and germination; discovery. EAST – WOOD.

The east is a good place for displaying photographs of your parents and other relatives, including your ancestors. You can honour your teachers and people whom you admire and learn from. The east is also well suited for books which stimulate new ideas. It is the area of initiation and healthy new growth with green as its dominant colour. Thriving plants, placed here in strong natural daylight, promote the life-long growth of fresh ideas and interests. Dried out wood will become rigid and snap while well-watered wood is flexible and forgiving. Remember to keep your own life fresh and vigorous.

The 4th Enrichment: fortunate blessings; abundance; prosperity; wealth; money; financial planning; budgeting; knowing what is enough for one's needs; generosity and altruism. SOUTH EAST – WOOD.

Symbolise abundance with a money plant [also known as a jade or friendship plant], the colour green [lime is vibrant], red ribbons tied through or around items you value, an aquarium, fish mobile, gorgeous shells, a water feature – whatever represents abundance for you. Keep this area totally free from clutter – if you are already 'full up' then you are not ready to receive. If the south east area of your plot or garden falls away too steeply, plant a strong tree or other retaining feature here.

The 5th Enrichment: physical health – your body, food, drink, exercise sleep, stress; mental and emotional well-being; whole life harmony; finding a balance; equanimity; honesty and personal responsibility. CENTRE – EARTH.

Always ensure that the centre of your home is absolutely gorgeous, clutter free, earthy and calm. Create a central area that encourages you to live well – the healthy interaction of mind and body as a single entity. You can make a placement as a reminder of the essential balance between life's ups and downs and the realisation that happy times are to be cherished and enjoyed. Paint a Yin-Yang symbol on a smooth pebble to illustrate the harmony between complementary opposites, creating a perfectly balanced whole. Display a bowl of earth objects to keep you 'grounded' yet ready to go out and cheerfully face the world. It is the area in which to focus on harmonious living. Our lives are inextricably linked to each other and to earth's bounties.

The 6th Enrichment: friendships; guides and helpful people; giving help to others; care for the environment; leisure and social life; travel and adventure; appreciation. NORTH WEST – METAL.

This is a good place to honour helpful friends by displaying their photographs or something they have given you. Gold and silver picture frames and metallic objects represent the robust nature of strong friendships and the potential for new bonds. A metal wind chime hung here brings helpful people into your life. If you like, place an animal or angel symbol to remind you of the unseen support of your sixth sense guides. The north west is also said to be favourable for energising opportunities for travel and adventure – display a world map or another appropriate symbol or picture. It is considered to be an area signifying strength in communion with others and in tune with the eco-system.

The 7th Enrichment: accomplishing creativity by bringing projects to fruition; overcoming procrastination; harvesting; celebration; relaxation; luck of children; family time; fun; surprises. WEST – METAL.

Celebrate your creativity and bringing projects to fruition in the west. This is the area where we applaud the transformation of ideas and harvest the outcome of our hard work. If you have a problem finishing things, then you can energise the west with a clock or another metallic motional object. Use white paint and décor to represent the potential of all colours and all things. Place reminders to encourage the 'harvesting' of your projects. In addition, celebrate children and playfulness here. It is also an ideal location for relaxing at the end of the day.

The 8th Enrichment: sanctuary; humanitarian and spiritual inquiry; belief; reflection; meditation; solitude; meaning and purpose; mortality; moral values and personal integrity; thanksgiving. NORTH EAST – EARTH.

This is a good place to site an easy chair and a bookcase, shelf or table for inspiring books and symbols – an amethyst crystal or a meditating Buddha – anything which helps you to 'think about thinking' and develop your inner being and contemplative nature. The north east is said to be the spiritual area. If you feel inclined, dedicate this as a sacred space and create a simple altar here – cover a small table with a beautiful cloth and adorn according to your beliefs. Purple is a regal colour that works well in this area but all gem colours and gems themselves are considered helpful – they are phenomenal products of the earth.

The 9th Enrichment: confidence in action; self-esteem; empowerment; expression; inspiration; motivation; recognition; significance; fame; shining your light; experiencing life to the full. SOUTH – FIRE.

Hang a crystal in a southern window – enjoy the radiating rainbows. Use their colour imagery and expansive energy to illuminate your self-development and capability to inspire others. Use splashes of red to energise yourself to action – whatever it takes to get you going – a vivid red flowering plant can invigorate your resolve. Too many representations of water in the south can kill your fire and dampen your resolve. Ideally you want to see, touch, hear, taste or smell objects or pictures that signify action. Burn candles or incense to fire yourself up and to boost your sense of self-worth. Use artificial lights if daylight is limited.

The Habitat Affect you create must feel 'right for you'

Please note that the Focus Feature suggestions above are just that – 'suggestions'. The most important determinant of how you create your Habitat Affect is that the resulting area or room appears gorgeous and stimulating to you, and to your family, if you live with other people. Therefore, in whatever area you choose to position a Focus Feature, simply ensure that its presence feels truly inspirational!

Five Focus Feature Factors

If you are planning to introduce Focus Features, the Five Factors below summarise a few of the more practical things you can do in support of your individual Habitat Affect.

[1] Visual appeal using paint

Add striking eye-catching appeal quickly to walls, ceilings, floors, windows and doors using paint colours that are appropriate to the function of the room. For spectacular results, use chalk paint [a brilliant relatively recent addition to your décor options], to give worn-out furniture a new lease of life. High lacquer gloss also looks good, while a satin finish revitalises tired kitchen units. Spray paint baskets, boxes, containers and other accessories for contemporary appeal. Let your chosen colours say something about you and the enrichment values you aspire to, rather than the latest interior design craze.

[2] Fabric appeal

From upholstery on sofas and chairs to cushions, curtains, blinds, tablecloths, towels and bed covers, fabric has a key visual and textual role to play in the feel of your home. Is it time for some uplifting new textiles in your life – maybe make a splash of bright bathroom towels, a new duvet-cover perhaps, a child-proof plasticised tablecloth, some sensual faux fur sofa cushions or a bold re-upholstered statement chair? How about a wall-hanging piece of fabric you found on holiday that reminds you of happy times? Do your fabrics enhance your personal Habitat Affect?

[3] Decorative extras and displays

Artworks in fabulous frames which tell an inspiring story? Photographs that cement relationships? Mood-enhancing wallpaper? Fancy wall lights? Do you love your wall displays? Barren or cluttered, do some of the items on your walls need a re-think? How about changing knobs or other inexpensive fixtures for a more personal feel? What about the extraneous objects on the various surfaces of your home – a vase of flowers, pot plants, ornaments, a fruit bowl, audio visual equipment, candles, books etc. You probably have a wide variety of 'things' surrounding you, but are they all necessary and do they all make you 'feel good'? Is it time for a cull of the old stuff with the possibility to introduce one or two new items to inspire you?

[4] The very best storage

Superb storage – easy to use and attractive – is key to a healthy household. What is your current situation as regards storing clothes, shoes, boots, hats, gloves – are your drawers, cupboards, shelves, hooks and rails adequate or do you need to add some? How about your kitchen units and dining storage, your recycling and waste disposal systems – are they good enough? Then there are the various items connected with your audio visual and e-life: smart phones, tablets, computers, chargers, back-ups, office stationary – are they stored in a practical way to aid efficiency? Similarly, think about your hobbies and storing all 'the stuff' you need to enjoy your leisure activities? Finally – what's hiding under the stairs or up in the attic? Review and renew your storage systems once in a while and life will become so much more pleasant and relaxed.

[5] Clutter watch – letting go

When was the last time you had a serious de-clutter? Remember the basics: if the item is no longer necessary for your present and future way of life, you can choose to recycle it, donate it to charity, sell it, 're-model' it to become useful again or throw it in the bin. Of everything you do retain, ensure that all essential moveable items have 'a storage home' within your home – this avoids the problem of clutter on surfaces: paper, clothes, makeup etc. Of everything more or less static in your home ask "does this make my heart sing?". If 'yes' it stays; if 'no' it goes; if 'not sure' probe the underlying reason for your hesitancy. When you find it difficult to 'let go' of something, ask yourself why? Acknowledging any such blockages, however challenging or possibly even painful, can be extremely useful for your personal development.

Refresh your Focus Features from time to time to reflect the person you aspire to be and always choose to make your surroundings a beautiful place to behold.

Be kind to yourself – make allowances

"Tenderness and kindness are not signs of weakness and despair but manifestations of strength and resolution." Kahlil Gibran. As you embrace the 9 Enrichments way of living, be sure to make allowances for difficulties and uncertainty. Personal kindness is key to your approach as there will always be days when things do not go according to plan. The worst thing you can do under these circumstances is to see yourself as a failure and abandon your journey.

Nobody is perfect and you would probably rank as a saint if you did not, on occasion, revert to some of the behaviour you are trying to unlearn. Good news! This is a prime opportunity for discovering a silver lining. Rather than self-disapproval, simply ask "what can I learn from this situation?"; whatever you glean from challenging yourself in this way will help to strengthen your resolve.

Review – to look back upon

Reviews without blame or judgement can be extremely enlightening. We give ourselves permission to look back upon how our life has been flowing. We make an assessment of what has been helpful and healthy and what has been unhelpful and unhealthy. We can benefit by acknowledging any poor choices that we may have made, without beating ourselves up, and identify the opportunities for change and growth within that particular area.

We can also acknowledge the fulfilling situations that have arisen and celebrate these.

Just occasionally you might like to ask yourself appropriate questions about each of your 9 Enrichments and how engaging with the Habitat Affect is helping you. You will intuitively know what it is you want to question because your life experience will be showing you where to focus attention.

Rewards

We like to emphasise that 'feeling good' about your life does not mean smug or complacent, rather it means experiencing the happy reward of 'joy' and 'enjoyment'. The more you feel at ease with yourself and your relationships with others, the more you will have to celebrate and be joyful about.

On top of these built-in rewards of well-being, remember to grant yourself occasional extra rewards – things that complement your choices-for-change. Your extra rewards can be anything from giving yourself time to read a book or do something charitable, to a meal out with friends, a special event, a long soak in the bath, a mountain hike, one night a week at dance class or …….. whatever you personally consider to be a bit of a treat.

It may sound unnecessary but building in regular rewards to honour your achievements is pretty vital. This is because they give positive confirmation to your endeavour and boost your enthusiasm for continuing year in, year out. Besides which, you can choose rewards that allow you to be 'playful'. And playfulness is one of the key energy states that many so-called 'grown-ups' have outgrown to their detriment. What sort of things would you like to reward yourself with? Can you think of a way to add rewards into your routine?

Making it happen

As you gradually put into practice the Habitat Affect changes you have identified as being valuable for living well, both your experience of the present and your upcoming life will benefit, as will everyone with whom you come into contact.

A hundred years from now it will not matter what my bank account was, the sort of house I lived in or the kind of car I drove – but the world may be a better place because I believed that, in my own small way, I could make a difference. So I will make it happen – whatever it is.

Appendix

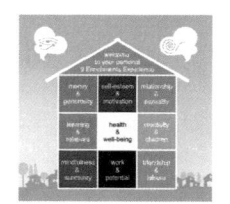

Appendix A: Colour attributes

As you might expect, colour is an extremely interesting and complex subject. Here we present a simplified description of various colours – a mix of science, western design and eastern mysticism – which you may find helpful for creating a supportive Habitat Affect in your home or workplace.

RED is associated with the fire element, warmth and summer. Red is the colour of alertness, movement and action. It is useful when you need to move energy around.

Red is perceived as a colour of strength. It is said to stimulate physical activity and vitality, feelings of self-esteem, confidence and recognition. Red is the colour of our blood, it represents life's nourishment, invigorating the body and feeding the mind with vital oxygen. Infrared is used to speed up the healing process.

Red can induce anger and aggression – the saying 'like red rag to a bull' has a firm psychological basis. So red is not advisable for hyperactive, violent or aggressive people. It is also unsuitable when relaxation is the priority for a particular room or area or garment.

Use red in rooms where activity is required. If you have a tendency to tire easily in the office – splashes of red objects or décor can help to keep you active.

We also use the term 'in the red' to denote financial problems. The red light is well known for its sexual connotations. Red is certainly a colour to use with care. The red heart symbol represents passionate love. If you want passion in your life make a gift of a red flower. Wear red accessories to embolden your appearance. Give someone you love a 'lucky' card or write a 'wish list' for yourself and place in a red envelope.

PINK is the softer more receptive tint or tone of red with earthen qualities. Pink is often associated with feminine values, peace-making and romantic love. It is the colour of gentle flowers and rose quartz crystals. Bright cerise pinks are daring, sexy and stimulating. Pale pinks are restful and calming. Pink can also be harmless and fun – pink elephants, the pink panther and Lily the Pink.

ORANGE is a mixture of fire and earth elements. It is sometimes known as the happiness colour and can also signify independence and optimism. Orange is said to govern your sexuality and physical performance. Use orange in playrooms, places for exercise and dance, and for social gathering areas where you can celebrate life. Avoid orange if you have an addictive personality. Wear orange for fun. Eat orange foods for vigour.

YELLOW is associated with the earth element, health, honesty and longevity. Yellow helps to centre us so that we are connected with our inner power. It has the capability to transform blue to green and red to orange. Likewise, it can help you to make transformative changes in your life while remaining grounded and receptive to reason.

Yellow is said to be the colour of knowing and communicating your intuitive 'gut feelings'. It stimulates mental clarity, verbal reasoning and will power. Use yellow in places of learning, where social gatherings take place and lively conversation is required.

Nature uses yellow for a variety of attractive flowers, but combines it with black to act as a danger signal. Do not use too much yellow if you are prone to stress and find it difficult to switch off mentally. Yellow is said to be related to the solar plexus chakra which links with our emotions – yellow is sometimes associated with fear, on the other hand sunshine yellow has a cheery quality which enlivens the spirit.

GREEN is associated with the wood element and spring. Green symbolises new growth and adaptability. It encourages flexibility in life without losing strength and stability – like a tree with its roots firmly grounded but swaying in the wind.

Green is the colour in the middle of the rainbow representing balance and it is said to promote positive feelings, compassion and sensitivity. Reputed to influence the heart and loving relationships, its reverse nature is linked to jealousy viz 'green with envy' and 'the green-eyed monster'. Happily, fresh lush green [think new grass], stimulates incoming ideas, creativity and the ability to accept change.

Use pale green in rooms where sensitivity is needed or where activities involve physical touch and healing. It is also good to emphasise family values and respect for family or community members. Avoid green in rooms where detached analytical thinking is required. Healthy plants are an ideal way to introduce green to indoor environments – ensure they are kept well-watered.

BLUE is associated with the water element and winter. Blue is the colour of mental reasoning, communication, principles and justice, and is said to promote altruism. It is linked with the throat chakra of eastern medicine. Pale blue is cool and calming while a bright electric blue is more stimulating – think of a clear blue sky that instantly brightens the spirit.

Blue light and blue surroundings are generally good for soothing the mind and dissipating headaches. Use blue in rooms where you want to relax like bedrooms and clinics but note: too much blue can make a room feel cold and isolated.

Blue features in sayings that reflect life's problems: 'I'm feeling blue' and 'playing the blues' whereas 'the blue ribbon' is a high honour and a rich cornflower blue makes people smile. Blue is also a 'safe' colour for blending in and is therefore recommended for business suits. Navy blue is popular for a non-confrontational demeanour and when a thoughtful appearance is required. Ubiquitous blue denim continues to appeal the world over.

PURPLE stimulates artistic and imaginative activities. It is associated with spiritual and psychic awareness. Purple combines the elements of fire and water in perfect balance. Purple can be used in moderation to inspire intuitive thought – the so-called sixth sense. It is particularly favourable in combination with silver indicating good fortune.

Use purple in rooms where you want to inspire aesthetic creativity or meditation. However, be warned that too much purple can lead to impracticality, day-dreaming and illusions. Purple is the colour of kings and is worn ceremonially to denote the highest authority. If you want to feel important, try a flash of purple.

BLACK is the total absence of colour and is associated with the water element. It represents your hidden potential and the possibility of all things on life's journey. 'Black as night' allows the potential for appreciating light – both metaphorically and in the form of celestial bodies. Danger, passion and risk are linked with black – yet without risk, life is stale.

Black can be sombre and black can denote evil but it can also be chic and very dramatic, especially in combination with white or silver. Too much black will make an area seem smaller – a useful tool for clothing. Black in combination with white gives us the distinctive yin-yang symbol conveying the idea of harmony between complementary opposites.

WHITE is associated with the metal element and autumn in eastern tradition. It symbolises the soul returning to the light when someone dies. White is the synthesis of all the other colours and is considered dynamic and vibrant. White enhances clear vision. It allows you to simplify your surroundings and gives you the single-mindedness to complete projects – the fruition of your creativity.

Too much white can give a stark appearance to a room which some people find unwelcoming. However, with the elegant use of pictures, objects and textiles, a mainly white décor can give a wonderful result.

Hang a crystal in a south facing window and see the white light being refracted into the colours of the rainbow that will reflect across your white walls. Allow the beam to focus on your 'middle eye' – think happily about the miracle of life that is 'you' – boosting your sense of well-being.

GREY – various tints of black with white are invaluable to artists for shading and creating perspective. Metaphorically grey is a useful colour for reminding us of our shadow side and that our perspective on the world need not necessarily be black and white – directly in opposition – but include shades of everything in between.

SILVER represents secret desires and intuition, particularly in combination with purple. Silver is precious and so are the spaces and objects which incorporate this metallic colour. The silvery moon is hypnotically special and seems to affect our psyche.

We sometimes refer to an eloquent speaker as having a silver tongue – meaning that their persuasive speech has the power to influence us. Ethnic silver jewellery has a distinctive quality which denotes a certain freedom of style.

GOLD is the colour of long-term ambitions, courage and wealth. Used subtly it signifies opulence and good taste. We talk about golden corn at harvest as we celebrate the bounty of the land. From ancient times, gold has been a cherished metal, fashioned into objects of desire – both golden coins and expensive jewellery. The gold wedding band is popular in many societies.

Gold features strongly in folk tales of alchemy but beware of lusting after gold – many people perished in 'the gold rush'. Golden light is uplifting while golden touches to décor – for instance picture frames or gold-sprayed accessories – can metaphorically 'gild the lily' [improve on whatever is already beautiful], in contemporary homes.

BROWN is nature's carpet of soil, fallen leaves and decaying matter – a solid earthy colour. It is the very ground on which man, animals and plants live – from the dirt floor to nutrient rich soils on which much of our food relies. While we suggest you use brown sparingly in your décor as it can be rather drab, it does signify a robust foundation so is good for floor coverings.

A brownish grey, used in moderation, can give a sophisticated look. Some of our most beautiful furniture comes in a variety of polished browns – mahogany, walnut, oak etc. – the range is wide. This is where brown can make a special statement in your home.

Brown wood fuels fire. Symbolically an ordinary static object – a dry log – is transformed into the extra-ordinary vibrant movement, heat and light of fire. Perhaps if we care to look deeply at the mundane ordinary things in our lives, we may see the potential for extra-ordinary experiences.

Appendix B: Dealing with fears, doubts and worry

If you choose to examine and face your fears, taking a positive 'choice-for-change' approach, you will be able to enjoy greater emotional freedom and also set a good example for others to follow.

Identifying your fears

True life-threatening fear aside, most of us have some irrational beliefs with their attendant fears which give us a distorted view of the world. These beliefs and fears may have been passed down from parent to child or have come from bad experiences that have resulted in feelings of guilt, resentment, shame or low self-esteem. Then there are the fears of those who find it difficult to cope with the demands of modern society or the worry generated by incessant media coverage of crime, natural disasters, medical problems – we are surrounded by scaremongers.

Some people hold onto unnecessary fears for years and years – sometimes for their entire life. If you feel like identifying a few of your own 'apparent' fears, here is a chance to take them out of your mental store cupboard one by one. Perhaps tell yourself that you are determined to expose and then banish any unnecessary fears.

As you identify your supposed fears, have a look at the reasoning behind them. You may find one or two of the questions below useful as a prompt. If your answer is 'yes' to any of the questions, think through your reasons for this fear and, if you feel like it, write a few words explaining your rationale. See if you can provide the 'because ……..'; for instance: "Yes – I'm afraid of being alone because ……..".

- ➢ Are you afraid of what other people may think or say about you?
- ➢ Are you afraid of failing to live up to some perceived ideal?
- ➢ If you are well, are you afraid of being seriously ill and dying?
- ➢ Are you afraid of getting older, particularly if you have reached 60?
- ➢ Are you afraid of taking risks? What sort of risks are you avoiding?
- ➢ Are you afraid of having inadequate financial means?
- ➢ Are you afraid of being unemployed?
- ➢ Are you afraid of the idea that you have done something wrong?
- ➢ Are you afraid of 'guilty' secrets being discovered?
- ➢ Are you afraid of …….. ask your own fear questions?

NB. If you are afraid of physical things such as heights, wide open spaces, confined spaces, fear of flying, spiders etc. you could choose to visit a professional working in hypnosis or systematic desensitisation [graduated exposure] therapy.

Thought-challenging your 'because …….. '

Have a look at the 'apparent' fear or fears that you feel relate to you and your 'because …. ' and do a spot of 'thought-challenging'. For each fear you have identified, challenge your current belief and think about 'the reality'.

Useful questions to answer are: What is it that I'm really afraid of here? Is my fear appropriate to the situation? In the worst case scenario, what is actually likely to happen? Can I see how my irrational beliefs are causing me to doubt myself and my abilities? What would be a realistic strategy for coping that neutralises my anxiety, doubt and worry? Can you see a common theme running through your fears: that the reality is usually far less serious than the fear?

Recollections

You can try using 're-collective logic' by remembering what actually happened last time this particular fear raised its ugly head in your life. Maybe the reality was nothing like as bad as the fear itself? Work with the rational sequence of events that did in fact take place and note your findings.

Of course, it may well be that you have uncovered a very real difficulty – let's say for example with your finances. Nonetheless by identifying it, and getting rid of the 'destructive' fear associated with it, you will subsequently be able to develop a 'constructive' plan for moving forwards [the 4th Enrichment Experience covers finances].

By deliberately facing your fears, challenging your negative thoughts and exposing the reasoning behind them, you enact your ability to change. Whatever your fear, the road to recovery and re-creation starts with 'acceptance'.

"May I have the courage today to live the life that I would love; to postpone my dream no longer, but do at last what I came here for – and waste my heart on fear no more." O'Donoghue.

Why worry?

Lots of people lose valuable hours in the grip of unnecessary fear that translates into highly emotional anxiety, doubts and worries – and nobody ever added even a minute of time to their life by worrying. How would you rather spend your time – worrying or not worrying? Could you refuse to worry? Could you refuse to harbour doubts?

By adopting a 'fear-less', 'worry-less', 'doubt-less' approach to life, you will actually feel more secure emotionally. Having emotional stability will, in turn, enable you to be more constructively practical and effective, even when surrounded by the challenges and difficulties that you are bound to encounter along life's eventful journey.

However please do not confuse our term 'fear-less' with 'fearless' as meaning 'reckless'. Throwing caution to the wind in the face of certain adversity is reckless. We are talking here about choosing helpful thoughts and actions that wipe out the needless fear that gives rise to hindering doubts and worries.

Create inner peace with emotional security

While there is every point in being realistic about problems and obstacles that inevitably arise equally, there is absolutely no point in worrying about them. Instead you can turn your time and energy to productive ways of dealing with difficulties and initiating change. Fortunately, there are effective methods to help you negate worries.

Do we all agree that 'thoughts need attention to survive'? [Post this saying in a prominent place for maximum impact.] When 'a worried thought' enters your chattering mind, you might normally give it your attention and go with it – the result will be that you reinforce the doubt or worry, and then worry some more.

The alternative is to use a simple mindfulness technique. When 'a worried thought' starts to plague your mind, just label it 'thought' and let it go. Then focus your mind on your breathing or chose to think about something else 'on purpose'. It could be something entirely different or it could be a useful way of finding a constructive solution for the difficulty that gave rise to the worried thought in the first place. If 'the worried thought' resurfaces [or any unnecessary destructive thought, for that matter], just repeat the labelling as 'a mere thought', and let it go.

This is a simple yet powerful exercise you can do anywhere, at anytime, for the rest of your life – the outcome can be pure emotional release as you no longer allow the worried thought to have a dominating hold over you.

Be an objective adviser

Another method for mitigating doubts and worries is to pretend you are someone else looking in from the outside at your problem as an unbiased observer. What would 'they' advise? Give yourself a pseudonym, physically sit in a different chair, put on someone else's shoes or wear a strange hat.

Now work out a constructive solution as an adviser to yourself, either in your mind or commit it to writing – see what happens. Needless doubts and worries will only remain if you have consciously or subconsciously chosen to leave their threatening cloud hanging over you. *"The practice of being an independent observer helps you stay stable and calm. It is the best way to approach a decision in any circumstance."* Enrique Simo.

Anything else hidden in your mental store cupboard?

There are other aspects of faulty thinking linked to irrational fears and beliefs that may hinder your progress. Playing the role of victim, feeling vaguely apprehensive a lot of the time which stymies decision-making, not knowing what you really want, behaving like a frozen rabbit trapped in the headlights, self-sabotage and excuses, all fall into this category.

It sounds perverse but states such as 'victimhood' and 'self-sabotage' can be subconsciously used to excuse the option of failing. For example: 'being too busy' to exercise regularly or 'being distracted' and not listening properly when someone is trying to communicate with you, or breaking a healthy eating diet because you are trying to lose weight too quickly and are therefore bound to fail.

There is a saying "you make your own luck" – it is also possible that you may unwittingly contribute to your own misfortune. It is helpful to understand the subtle ways in which you behave, give out signals to others, lack focus or make excuses. You may not be immediately conscious of all the nuances that go to make up a particular situation, so you may need to delve deep. This is by no means a negative exercise; it is extremely liberating to know that you have the power to stop the sabotage of your intentions by recognising and dealing with the situation in an intelligent way.

Challenge your particular demons

Again, it can be useful to ask: what's my 'because' ……..? You can answer this by selecting one or two of the 'because' sentences below that strike a chord with you, and finish them with whatever you believe is really going on:

> I feel like I am the victim of circumstance because ……..
> I accept life isn't always fair, nevertheless I sometimes say 'it's not fair' or something similar because ……..
> I'm actually making my situation worse because …….
> I'm hindering myself by hiding my feelings because …….
> I'm not admitting the true picture to myself because ……..
> The reason I think …….. or do …….. is because ……...

Have a think about your current 'because reasoning'. What can you learn from this?

Your beautiful chest of drawers exercise

This exercise presents you with a thoughtful tool for dealing with fears, doubts and worries by putting them into perspective – be they past, present or future.

Start by getting into a comfortable position either sitting or lying down. In your imagination, bring into being **a beautiful chest of drawers**. It is your secret chest where you keep your innermost thoughts. It has three drawers.

The bottom drawer is where you can store all your past influences – it is where all your memories, good and bad, can be kept until you are ready to say goodbye to them forever. It is where some of your outmoded habits reside; it is where certain emotions live on, neatly tucked away but still accessible if you decide to show them.

The middle drawer is where you can store your present 'worries'. Once in the drawer you can begin to see that there is nothing to be gained by worrying. All you do is to increase your own stress triggers, anxiety and panic levels. There is however everything to be gained from being realistic and constructive about your present position. Even those things that you believe to be your biggest problems can present you with opportunities for change and refreshment – see if you can spot them.

The top drawer is where you can put any concerns you may have about the future – safely and tidily shut away from your everyday experience. The fact is that nobody has a certain future, uncertainty is the breath that keeps life interesting. Worrying about something that does not even exist – the future – is the biggest waste of time ever. It can also be very depressing. Instead, turn your top drawer storage into ideas about what you want to create for the future and how you can constructively bring these into play. Your drawer can store these constructs as useful items that can be changed as often as you want.

Your mental store cupboard

You can use your chest of drawers as an imaginary mental store cupboard for most aspects of your life. It allows you to visualise taking items out from time to time, acknowledging them and then either throwing them away forever or putting them back in the drawer for a future airing.

When you take them out for a good think, you may decide that, before you replace them in the drawer, you will change their appearance. This could be likened to re-packaging them – making them easier to understand next time.

For example, you may feel that part of your childhood was disturbing. Having a designer drawer allows you to acknowledge this but, instead of letting it ruin your day-to-day existence now, you can mentally 'put it into a closed drawer'. When you feel ready, you can take it out and examine it, possibly with the help of a friend or therapist. You could decide that it is no longer part of your life today and mentally throw it away or burn it. If you are not ready to discard it completely, because part of you still needs the prop of your past, however unpleasant, then try to give it a new wrapping of understanding. That means viewing it in a different way before putting it back in the drawer. Next time you take a look, your understanding will be truer.

Physical version

If you actually like the idea of physically writing down the items you want to store – past memories, present difficulties, future concerns – you can keep them in a three-drawer plastic or cardboard mini-chest, the type available from home or office storage departments. This hands-on physical involvement with decision making – rethinking or sometimes completely discarding items – is a powerful interactive tool.

"Today I will know that I don't have to worry about anything. If I do worry, I will do it with the understanding that I am choosing to worry, and it is not necessary!"

Appendix C: Inside the elements

Quantum physicists and cosmologists look at the world with extra dimensions. For instance, take the familiar observable world and factor in the fourth dimension of space-time, now nothing is as it seems to the 'logical' human 3D mind. Without an understanding of space-time, Einstein's theory of relativity would not stand up to scrutiny and many of today's brilliant technologies, of which we all take advantage, would not exist.

If you want to get a little technical for a moment, underpinning the extreme intricacy of the universe are the elements – you are doubtless familiar with the names: carbon, hydrogen, oxygen, calcium, sodium, potassium, iron, copper, tin etc. In fact, so far, 118 elements have been discovered – 92 from nature, the remainder have been made in laboratories. If you are interested, you can see the Periodic Table of Elements on the internet for more detail.

An element is 'a substance that cannot be separated into simpler components by chemical means' and each has specific chemical properties. Every element has a distinct atomic number – this is the number of protons in the nucleus of one atom which is equal to the number of electrons associated with that atom. If you could see inside the individual atoms of an element, you would find a host of sub-elemental entities [waves and particles]. These are the fundamental building blocks of matter, light and all energetic processes.

It is worth emphasising that everything in the universe, including us, is composed of these interactive sub-atomic entities – electrons, protons, neutrons, quarks, leptons, photons [quanta of light], bosons etc. [the Higgs boson being a popular subject at the moment having recently been discovered at CERN].

Paradoxically, at this sub-nuclear level, there is simply the perpetual motion of energy transfer. Einstein's famous equation $E=mc2$ shows that energy and matter [wave and particle] have an inseparable equivalence. He tells us that: *"Mass and energy are both but different manifestations of the same thing – a somewhat unfamiliar conception for the average mind"*. Our sun, from which all the available energy on earth originates, is a giant nuclear fusion machine relying on the perpetual motion of the elemental waves and particles within hydrogen atoms. A slightly daunting thought.

Hopefully, with this information, you can now go some way towards appreciating that everybody and everything on the planet, and in the universe, is part of this interdependent never-ending cycle of energy exchange. This may seem quite obtuse to the way you live your everyday life, nevertheless, it is humbling to realise the sheer brilliance of the universe 'out there' which is intricately linked to 'in here' – the very nature of your own consciousness.

Appendix D: Mindfulness practice – an overview

Mindfulness meditation has its roots in Buddhism and the idea that your mind is both the source of confusion that causes your suffering and the source of your potential transformation to enlightened living. However, you can benefit from practicing mindfulness whether or not you have any knowledge of Buddhism. In fact, today, as well as private meditation classes, mindfulness techniques are being employed in the workplace to create a more productive 'mindful' environment and in clinical therapeutic settings to help people with mental health issues.

Practicing mindfulness involves taking a look behind the scenes, as it were, of your own consciousness with the aim of learning to 'see things as they really are'. If you are interested in trying mindfulness meditation for yourself, you will find detailed instructions in the Action Area of the 8th Enrichment Experience: ACTION C: Thoughts – let them go!

As you come to understand the nature of your own mind, you gain insight into the causes and conditions of your day-to-day 'suffering' – those dramas, problems and worries that take up so much of your time and energy. You may find that your 'suffering' is most often the result of your very own emotions, thoughts and actions, as they manifest within your personal, social and cultural circumstances.

The suffering created by attachment

A prime cause of suffering, according to Buddhist teaching, is 'attachment'. As you mature, you become attached to certain habits and beliefs, to people and to material things – way more than you actually need for survival and for happiness. These attachments can often last for years when they are no longer appropriate. In order to rid yourself of obstructive attachments and desires, it is helpful to think about impermanence – that everything changes over time – no exceptions.

To break out of the cycle of suffering and experience well-being, there are 7 basic principles:

- focus on experiencing the present moment
- be 'mindful' of your thoughts and emotions
- quieten your chattering mind
- think before you act and be skilful in your speech
- discriminate without being prejudiced or judgemental
- refrain from harmful actions
- show kindness and compassion towards others.

Being 'mindful' allows you to calmly acknowledge and accept 'what is' and then choose an appropriate response – either action or non-action – which releases you from the suffering of worry and the worry of suffering! If you think about it, most of the stuff that you worried about in the past probably didn't happen anyway, or certainly not in the way that you expected.

The rewards of mindfulness

The skill of single-pointed mindfulness is extremely useful for your everyday life. By training your mind, you learn how to stop your 'chattering monkey mind' from taking over which allows you to give 100% attention to the things that really matter. If a thought that is likely to hinder or damage you arises – as it surely will many times over – you can simply label it 'thought – let it go'. This really works and you will find, over time, that the process of 'letting go of your thoughts' becomes second nature to you.

How often you meditate and for how long at any one session is entirely up to you. Do not be put off by books or even people you know suggesting you need to meditate for long periods, if this is unsuitable for you. It is better to establish a routine you can keep up, rather than start with an unrealistic regime that is unsustainable with your daily lifestyle. Five to ten minutes every morning, or whenever it suits you, is a reasonable way to start. Alternatively, you might try 'walking meditation' during your lunch hour – say ten minutes or so while you walk around your local park.

You will notice after only a few days of meditating, that you feel more alert. Strangely, you may also find that you seem to have more time! Maybe this is because you are more efficient and smarter at prioritising. The few minutes a day meditating seems to give you 'a time bonus' pay back, quite apart from the health benefits and the helpful energy that you exude to those around you.

Appendix E: Ready to receive

This is the story of an apparently successful man called Mr. Too and his experience upon consulting the wise teacher Master How-So.

Mr. Too was very clever and wealthy but he was also arrogant, discontent and desperately wanted to find 'the secret of a happy life'. He decided to consult a local teacher who was reputed to be very astute and happy.

Mr. Too was pleased to be invited to Master How-So's modest house for tea. Once seated, Mr. Too inquired "Master How-So, I have come to learn how to have a happy life, please can you tell me?"

Master How-So smiled gently without speaking and slowly proceeded to pour Mr. Too a cup of tea. The warm green liquid reached the top of the cup but, to Mr. Too's amazement, Master How-So continued to pour the tea until it started to overflow into the saucer.

Mr. Too looked on in disbelief. At the point where the tea began to flow onto the tray, he politely pointed out that the tea was spilling. However, Master How-So didn't appear to register and still continued to pour.

Eventually the tea flooded the table and then overflowed to the floor. At this point Mr. Too jumped to his feet aghast and grabbed the tea pot from Master How-So. Mr. Too was amazed that Master How-So just sat there smiling.

After a short pause the wise teacher said "Now you have your answer Mr Too. If you are too full up, there is no room for anything else – no room for you to experience the happiness you already have within. When you are given opportunities to change, they overflow and are wasted!"

As Mr. Too took his leave, he bowed his head and profusely thanked Master How-So. Now Mr. Too understood the importance of being ready to receive. From that day on he determined to abandon his arrogant know-it-all persona and live a humbler life in the service of others – almost immediately Mr Too began to experience what it feels like to be happy.

Appendix F: Keeping love alive

10 golden guidelines – well worth the effort

- You both made the choice to spend your 'life-time' with each other so, if things are not brilliant between you, go back in your mind to a time when everything was wonderful and work out how to re-create this together. Talk constructively – this means being honest about what you would like to happen now and then choose what you both need to do to make this happen. And always remember that 'actions speak louder than words'.

- Never take each other for granted. Show your appreciation for the little things, as well as the grand gestures, on a daily basis. Make sure you say 'thank you' and 'I love you' frequently and mean it. If you find yourself not meaning it, then do some serious heart-searching and nip any problems in the bud before they become entrenched.

- How about a weekly discussion at a mutually suitable time – a diarised appointment you always try to keep? You need to make a prior agreement that both of you can talk openly about whatever issues may be niggling you – without fear of giving offence – because having this discussion is for the very best of the relationship. Always try to be diplomatic and constructive in the way you phrase things – skilful speech. At the same time, you can offer praise or thanks for all the good things that you have experienced recently. This can be a helpful way to avoid major arguments and cement your commonality.

- Try to do activities together – particularly the ones that brought you together in the first place – or experience the excitement of jointly planning to try something new. When you are making arrangements to do things with other people, always have the courtesy to check diaries so your partner feels included in your plans, even if he or she will not be present. When last minute requests – family, friends, business or community matters – arrive unexpectedly, be tolerant of a change of plan, as long as it is reasonable and infrequent.

- If you find yourself gossiping about your partner's faults to other people, then it is time to review what is going on in your mind. Love is not present in idle chatter – only say things you would be happy to repeat directly to your partner. We are each responsible for the words that come out of our mouth and, assuming you want to stay in the relationship, your speech needs to create and sustain a climate of consent for joy in partnership.

- Surprises and adventures are quite important from the beginning but especially so after you have been together for several years. It is all too easy to get stuck in a rut. Having 'a surprise date night' once a month is a great way to keep a relationship 'alive'. You can alternate as organiser – so that makes six surprise dates a year each – not really that onerous when you think about it. If you prefer to be more spontaneous, just ensure that your spontaneity refrains from slip sliding away with the passing years.

- Disparity over money and finances is notorious as a problem generator. To keep love alive and untainted by economic argument, make sure this is an area you are prepared to discuss openly, brushing it under the carpet never helps in the long run. If your personal finances are out of parity, it is important to accept this and agree on a joint strategy for dealing with household and family expenses. However, if one or both of you, is spending too much on unnecessary items or has an expensive addiction, then it may be time to seek professional help.

- Keep up appearances – it is easy to slop around at home in unappealing clothes with lack of attention to grooming. Try, within reason, to present yourself as you did when you were attracting your partner during the early phase of your relationship. As for the bedroom, if wearing sexy underwear boosts your self-confidence then do it for yourself and not because you feel coerced. Ladies – learn to love your 'wobbly bits'! If you feel good about yourself, you are more inclined to enjoy love-making which will be of benefit to your partner as well.

- Be a hand-holding, hugging, snuggler. Holding hands when you are out on a walk is a great gesture of 'togetherness'. When you are coming and going from home separately, always try to acknowledge your partner with a kiss or a hug. When you are watching TV, snuggle up together. These are all simple little physical things at the heart of a loving relationship.

- Frequently smile at each other, laugh, have fun. Really look at your partner with your eyes wide open when he or she is talking to you, listen carefully to what they are saying and respond with loving kindness. Finally: 'never let the sun go down on your anger' – a well-known saying it pays to remember from time to time.

Appendix G: Appreciating the miracle of me

Before embarking on this imaginative bodily appreciation, please note that the description below is necessarily general and typical. If you are reading this and have a physical disability, please adapt the wording to suit your body. We acknowledge that all bodies are wonderful in their own individual way and, in particular, the tremendous ability that we have for adapting in atypical scenarios.

A journey through myself

In my mind's eye, I am taking a journey through myself. I view my body as an extra-ordinary living working organism – a consumer of foods and drinks, a physical performer, a sexual being, an enjoyer of comfortable and aesthetically pleasing surroundings. I am blessed with a rich variety of physical ways in which to interact with the people, the creatures, the objects and the energy of this world.

I have five major sensory organs – my eyes, my ears, my nose, my tongue and my skin. Through these I sense things I sometimes take for granted – the marvel of sight, sound, smell, taste and touch.

I have bones and muscles enabling me to move my body parts in a huge variety of ways. I have strong arms ending in my incredible hands that allow me to carry out an enormous number of actions, everything from holding and manipulating objects to hugging my nearest and dearest. I have robust legs ending in complex ankles and feet so I can stand upright and walk and run and jump and pedal.

I have a voice box which means I can produce recognisable sounds when I talk or sing. I have two magnificent spongy organs called lungs that allow me to bring oxygen into my body and get rid of waste carbon dioxide. I have the ability to produce liquids which means I can cry, I can lubricate my mouth, my nasal linings and my sexual organs. I have an ever-beating heart, the central pump of an ultra-efficient system for transporting blood around my body to provide nourishment for my cells and to fight disease. When I injure myself, my blood has the ability to clot and allow the wound to heal over.

My digestive system is quite phenomenal in the way it handles so many different types of food and liquids, what's more, it has to do this regularly around two, three or even four times every single day. The same relentless routine goes for my waste disposal systems to rid my body of noxious materials. Excretion involves several intriguing processors – my filtering kidneys and my bladder, my lower bowel and rectum, plus a bit of help from my sweating skin and my lungs for gaseous waste.

Then there is my endocrine system producing the hormones that regulate, and act as catalysts for a multitude of bodily functions. It is thanks in part to these bio-chemicals, and to the wonderful gift of sex, that I and my partner can create another human being who will have half my genetic characteristics and half those of my mate. All in all, it's an amazing body I've got here – I really am quite remarkable!

But that's not it by any means. I have a brilliant nervous system which links all my body parts and allows most everything to work in harmony. Above all this, I have an awesome physical brain – an undulating lump of grey matter. My brain is my star mental performer allowing me to experience my body's physicality and to interpret the signals from my sense organs. Most fascinating of all, my brain allows me to think, to create ideas, to sleep, to dream, and to make sense of the world in which I live.

Hello brain – it's thanks to you that I can follow this journey through myself and ask the big questions. Am I really just a body with a brain? Surely there's more to it than that? So what controls my brain? I do! Who am I? What am I? Am I my mind?

My mind allows my experiences through the medium of my brain. I like to think that my mind has choice, although I do not always exercise that choice. In fact, sometimes I fail to recognise that my mind is really the power behind the throne, so I just let my body, my unchallenged emotions and external events dictate what I do. In this way, I neglect to give my physical body the mental respect it deserves.

On occasion, I react to circumstances and abandon good sense. So today the plan is to learn a better way of being – to know my own mind, to override my emotions and to stay focused – my mind chooses my thoughts and actions appropriately. But am I just my mind? What about my soul, my spirit, my higher self, my Buddha nature, my Atman essence? My spirit keeps my mind wondering . . .

Appendix H: Foods and vitality

Foods to boost your energy levels – just a few examples
[in alphabetical, rather than nutritional, order]

- ✔ Avocados
- ✔ Beans – sprouting, dried, frozen, occasionally canned
- ✔ Bread made of wholegrain flour – wheat, rye, oats etc
- ✔ Cereals – porridge, oatmeal, wholegrain wheat etc; check for added fats and sugars
- ✔ Dried fruit – apricots, prunes, sultanas, figs
- ✔ Fresh fruit – apples, pears, kiwis, oranges, bananas, blueberries, pineapples, melons, figs, plums, cherries
- ✔ Fresh and frozen vegetables – all types – masses to choose from including seaweed
- ✔ Herbs of all kinds – you can grow them in pots
- ✔ Honey – good quality in small quantity
- ✔ Lentils and all legumes – peas, runner beans etc
- ✔ Nuts – unsalted – almond, brazil, cashew, walnut etc
- ✔ Oily fish – salmon, mackerel, herring
- ✔ Olives and olive oil used in moderation
- ✔ Pasta – wholegrain – avoid high fat sauces
- ✔ Seeds – sunflower, sesame, pumpkin, linseed – prepare in coffee grinder just before use

- ✔ Soya milk – unsweetened – other non-dairy 'milks'
- ✔ Yam – sweet potato – ordinary potatoes – avoid high fat cooking methods and accompaniments
- ✔ Yogurt – natural with live bacteria cultures

Foods which may deplete your energy levels and well-being

- ✘ All highly refined foods – white flour, white sugar, cakes, biscuits, sweets, etc
- ✘ All highly processed foods
- ✘ Anything unnatural
- ✘ Foods cooked in plastic containers
- ✘ Foods which contain modified fats
- ✘ Foods which contain certain artificial additives
- ✘ Foods which contain artificial colouring
- ✘ Most chocolate and sweets
- ✘ High fat/high sugar ice-cream
- ✘ Too much caffeine eg. coffee, strong tea, cola drinks
- ✘ Too much alcohol – especially on an empty stomach
- ✘ Unnecessary fat added to your food – taste the bread!
- ✘ Sugary drinks of all types
- ✘ Diet drinks with lots of additives

Appendix I: Developing your listening skills

When it comes to developing and maintaining friendships or working effectively in a team, listening intently is a crucial part of two-way communication. It also heightens awareness of the world around you. 'Hear and Now' is a workshop module we designed some years ago – we summarise it here to help you improve your listening skills.

Listening facts

The average person spends nearly three quarters of their waking time engaged in one of the four types of 'communication' – listening – talking – reading – writing. However, during our formal education, reading and writing skills are emphasised. The skills of speaking and, most importantly, listening are not always highlighted to the same extent. Because listening plays a vital role in everyday communications, it affects everything we do and expect to be done. There are three principle ways in which we listen – socially, naturally, internally.

Socially – listen to other people talking

Do you make a conscious effort to hear and understand the speech of others? Recall [a] the last time you really listened to someone with 100% focus, and [b] the last time, as far as you are aware, you didn't give your full listening attention to someone. What do these examples teach you, if anything? Was [a] a conscious choice? Was [b] a conscious choice?

Maybe try a spot of role play with a friend and take turns to discuss a topical subject or describe a set object.

APPENDIX

Then, after an agreed period of time, see how much of each other's part of the conversation, you can both recall. Of course, in this case you are primed to listen, but the experience may help you for future 'un-primed' listening opportunities.

Naturally – listen to the sounds of the physical environment

Do you make a conscious effort to experience the exciting sense and sensation of hearing 'natural' and 'aesthetically-created' sounds – music – birdsong – water – wind – bells etc? Most of us could benefit from spending more time enjoying the sounds from our physical environment. Next time you go for a walk in nature, close your eyes for a while and listen. When you listen to music, try and differentiate between the various musical instruments and harmonies or discords that make up the whole composition.

Internally – listen to the dialogue in your mind

Do you actively take the time to check your own thoughts and maybe have an internal conversation? Checking our thoughts and being a mindful observer are skills that eastern religions emphasise. 'Internal listening' can bring us fresh insight to our circumstances, attitude, mood and behaviour.

Ideas for ways to improve your listening skills

- Bring listening into your conscious mind whenever it is appropriate.

- Fix your mind onto what the other person is saying and the messages they are trying to convey. Their tone of voice and body language will also give you clues as to what they are really trying to say.

- When you are listening to someone who is not physically present – for example on the telephone – ensure you are not distracted by your computer screen or a doodle pad, unless doodling aids concentration!

- Try not to 'half listen' as you prepare your own rejoinder. Refrain from being too ready to jump in with your own speech. A considered response is far more skilful than an instant reaction.

- Do a 'thinking – listening' assessment when you have a moment on your own. First clear your mind of unnecessary clutter. Then ask yourself what gives you the most pleasure during social interactions – is it talking about yourself, is it hearing what other people have to say or is it the buzz of a stimulating two-way conversation? If you like the sound of your own voice too much, then it is time to develop your listening skills.

- Take a walk outside every day and commune with nature. Still your thoughts and concentrate on the sounds or absence of sounds inside and around you. With practice the part of your character that listens and interprets wisely will be you – most of the time. The philosopher Nietzsche is reputed to have said: "All truly great thoughts are conceived while walking."

- Here's a great maxim for listening: it is said that the wise person speaks only when they can improve on the silence – shhhhhhh!

Appendix J: From flour to flourishing

First you need a passion for a particular kind of bread, then you can develop a recipe or start with someone else's basic recipe and personalise it. Next you assemble the ingredients and put in the work. This involves actively mixing and kneading and a passive period while the yeast multiplies.

You have various choices as to how you shape the dough – smooth or platted, circular or rectangular – whether you produce one large loaf or several smaller buns, whether you finish the top with added seeds or leave it plain. You put the dough in a warm place and it rises slowly ready for baking.

You have pre-heated the oven, so now you set the timer and leave the bread to bake until the timer pings. You test the bread to see if it is ready or not. You do this by tapping the bottom to hear if there is a hollow sound. Still too doughy? Then you may need a little extra oven time.

You invite your family or friends to share in the eating of the bread. At this point you feel pretty good – it's that sense of achievement about the creative process you've just been through as demonstrated by your freshly baked bread. The word philosophers sometimes use for this feel-good factor is 'flourishing'. Seeing your creative bread-making project through to completion has allowed you to flourish.

Unfortunately, procrastinators are unlikely to experience the wondrous sense of achievement that accompanies a job well done – rising to a challenge, creating a solution and finishing the project – metaphorically they fail to bake their perfect loaf.

The ingredients for freedom from procrastination

By using the task-based ingredients below to harness your creativity, you can succeed in bringing projects to fruition.

- Know your creative passions – these are the areas to develop.
- Have a 'can-do' attitude – it puts a positive complexion on most things.
- Develop a talent for spotting opportunities and investigating hunches.
- Involve like-minded people if it feels right to collaborate.
- Express your overall goal which needs to embrace a 'do-able' journey.
- Be very clear about the constituent tasks required on the journey and specifically identify each one.
- Diarise a time schedule for dealing with each task.
- Be prepared to put in the time and effort with focus, hard work and enjoyment.
- Recognise unnecessary distractions as they arise, some will be very appealing – avoid them at all costs.
- Be open to making minor changes for best results – but avoid time-wasting by going off on a tangent.
- Give yourself a mini-reward each time you conclude a particular task.
- Celebrate the final completion of your project in style.
- Be grateful for your capability to finish a project and encourage others to use their creative talents well.
- Within the realm of reason, whatever you want to achieve – tell yourself "I can do it" – because you can!

Appendix K: Reality and your choices

Ask yourself: 'What does the human brain – my brain – do?'. It processes neurological stimuli – the 'data' we continually perceive physically and conceive mentally. It somehow converts this neurological data into thoughts – ideas and concepts – that can be expressed physically in language and through bodily actions. Then there is the mind.

'What does the human mind – my mind – do?' It uses these thoughts – ideas and concepts – as 'information'. It often deals with these concepts as if they represent reality. But they are merely our thoughts – our ideas about reality – often about how we want reality to be. Therefore the mind does not actually process reality as a universal truth but our individual version of it to suit our personal life story.

In other words, our perceptions, beliefs and emotional feelings shape our ideas about reality. In this way, we actually create a concept that we call 'reality'. Insomuch as we create our own reality, we have the power to create 'a reality' that suits our purpose, and the purpose of other sentient beings, on this earth at this time and in this place.

So what are the choices? We can choose to embrace the idea of living life with purpose and meaning. Our purpose is daily to acknowledge this precious life we have been given on earth and to use it well. Our life 'well-lived' is about making the most of our innate talents, our learned skills and the gifts of love and compassion, so we meet both our own physical and mental needs, and the needs of others with whom we interact.

Appendix L: Compass-element chart

SOUTH EAST WOOD 4th Enrichment	SOUTH FIRE 9th Enrichment	SOUTH WEST EARTH 2nd Enrichment
fortunate blessings; abundance; prosperity; wealth; money; financial planning; budgeting; knowing what is enough for one's needs; being generous; altruism.	self-esteem; confidence; motivation; action; empowerment; fame; expression; inspiration; recognition; shining your light; significance; experiencing life fully.	personal relationships; love; romance; sexual intimacy; compromise; companionship; the joy of sharing; contently single; looking for a like-minded soulmate.
EAST **WOOD** **3rd Enrichment**	**CENTRE** **EARTH** **5th Enrichment**	**WEST** **METAL** **7th Enrichment**
life-long learning; curiosity; engaging new ideas; personal growth; respect for parents, ancestors, teachers, coaches and leaders; initiation; discovery.	health; body image, food, alcohol, exercise, sleep, stress; mental and emotional well-being; harmony; finding a balance; equanimity; honesty; responsibility.	creativity – bringing projects to fruition; disabling procrastination; harvesting; celebration; relaxation; family time; luck of children; fun; surprises.
NORTH EAST **EARTH** **8th Enrichment**	**NORTH** **WATER** **1st Enrichment**	**NORTH WEST** **METAL** **6th Enrichment**
sanctuary; humanitarian and spiritual inquiry; belief; faith; reflection; meditation; solitude; meaning; mortality; moral values; integrity; thanksgiving.	work; career; vocation; volunteering; using your skills; releasing hidden potential; consolidation of ideas; planning; hibernation; the seed waiting in the ground.	friendships; guides and helpful people; giving help to others; care for the environment; leisure and hobbies; socialising; travel and adventure; appreciation.

Appendix M: The 5 elements

THE 5 ELEMENTS: EARTH - METAL - WATER - WOOD – FIRE

In traditional oriental building design, the compass directions were associated with the 5 elements. Oriental medicine is also based on these elements. Your personal 'Habitat Affect' can be enhanced by using the 5 elements symbolically to create Focus Features in your home to remind you of your aspirations and enrichment choices.

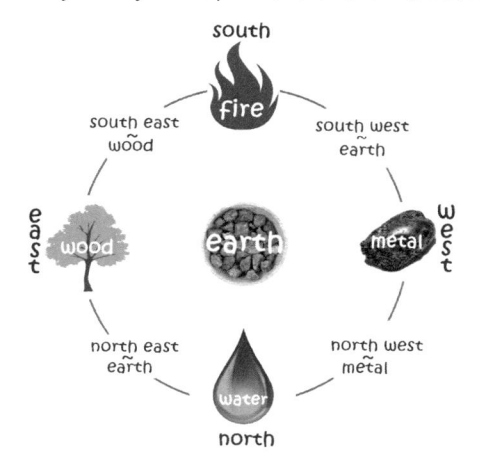

```
                          south
                          fire
         south east              south west
           wood                    earth

    e                                        w
    a      wood      earth      metal        e
    s                                        s
    t                                        t

         north east              north west
           earth                   metal
                          water
                          north
```

EARTH: represented by stones, rocks, pebbles, gems, soil, sand, gravel, ceramics, earthy pictures, yellow objects, yellow décor.

METAL: represented by metal objects, metal furniture, saucepans, TV, computers, pictures featuring metal, white/silver/gold décor.

WATER: represented by water feature, fountain, bowl of water, fish tank, glass objects, pictures of water, black/blue objects and décor.

WOOD: represented by living plants and trees, wooden furniture, pictures of plants, trees and green subjects, green objects and décor.

FIRE: represented by lights, candles, incense burning, fireplace, red objects, pictures featuring fire or red subjects, red décor.

THE END

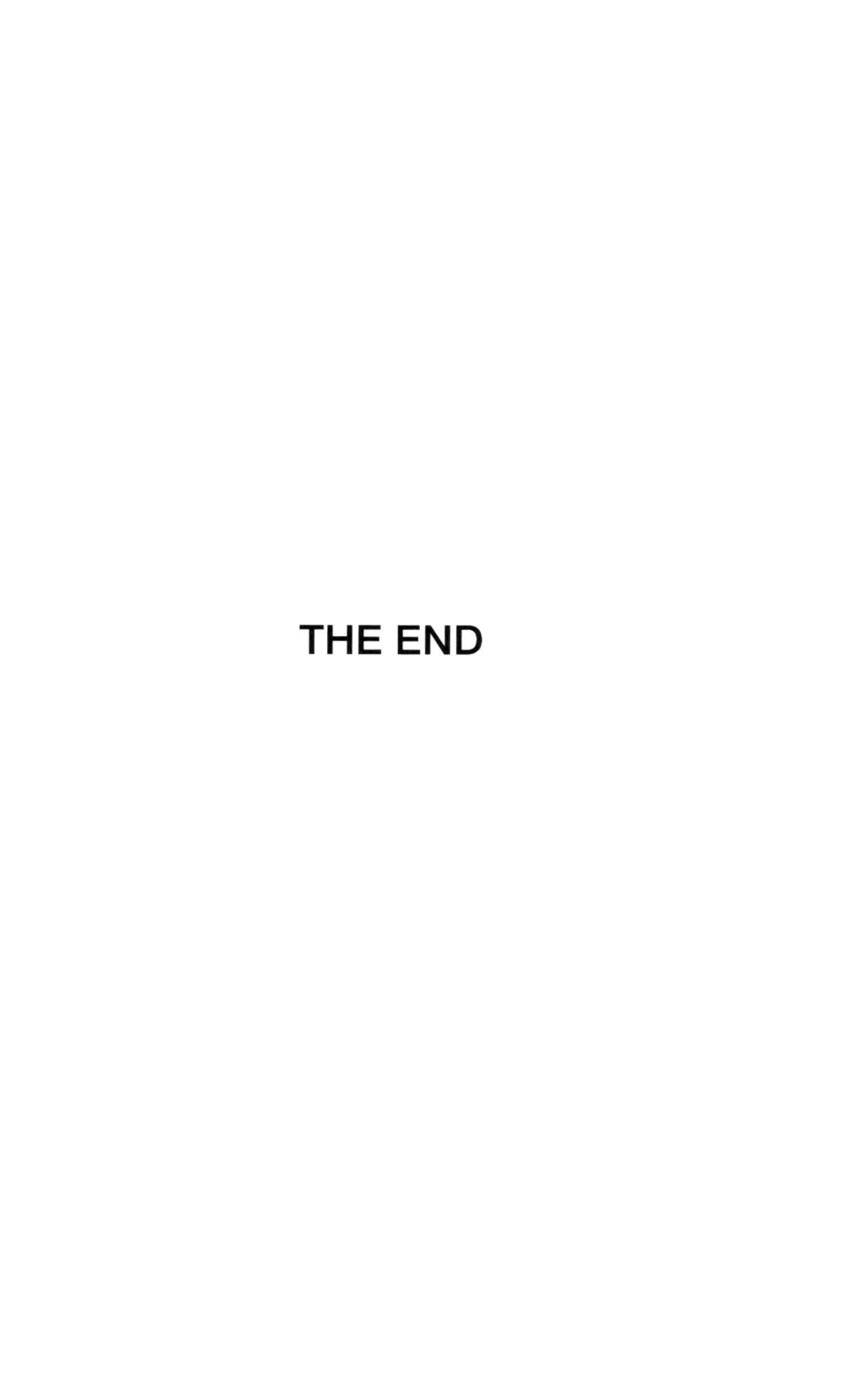

ABOUT THE AUTHOR

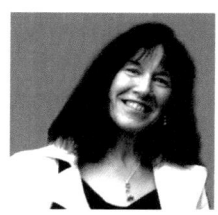

Anna Cherry is a BSc Psychology Graduate [Bristol] with a keen interest in the psychology of mindfulness and environmental influences. A former regional PR Director for a global advertising agency, Anna subsequently established an independent Communications Consultancy specialising in building design, construction materials, fire safety, acoustics and energy conservation. During this time, she authored numerous articles for technical publications and lobbied government regarding building regulations.

Linking her knowledge of buildings with a Diploma in Feng Shui [Holistic Design Institute], Anna has advised individuals and businesses on how their environment affects their lives and productivity. In similar vein, she developed a series of successful workshops [Clutter-busting, Feng Shui Introduction, Psychology of Place, Personal Potential, Listening Skills, Stress Address] and has been guest speaker at business clubs, along with TV appearances. Through her interest in Buddhist ethics, she was invited to be consultant editor, providing secular interpretation, for the 1st edition of '16 Guidelines for a Happy Life', based on the teachings of a 7th century Tibetan Emperor. Anna's hobbies include racket sports, hiking in nature, reading, sewing, DIY and socialising with friends. She lives near Oxford and regularly visits family in London, Spain and California.

Consultant Editor – Chloe Roberts

After graduating from Oxford University (BA Hons PPE), Chloe spent five years in India studying Tibetan Buddhism under great masters such as His Holiness the Dalai Lama and His Holiness Karmapa. She has been a student of the Karmapa ever since and recently organised his first trip to the UK in May 2017.

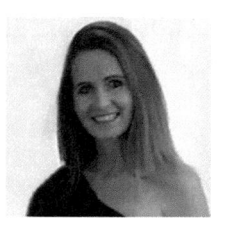

Passionate about the power of the mind, Chloe believes that individuals and organisations can become much more focused, compassionate and dynamic by looking at the mind and its capabilities. It is this belief that drives her management style when developing and nurturing a team of over 50 staff across offices in LA, NYC and London in her role as Executive Vice President for a global entertainment company. Chloe's understanding of the value of mindfulness, of maintaining a work-life balance, and of working smart, rather than hard or fast, not only infuses the day-to-day company working ethos but also ensures she can be a hands-on mother of two. Ever resourceful, while on maternity leave, Chloe invented 'LapBaby' – an innovative hands-free baby product now stocked worldwide.